Rest, Recover, Rise

ENOUGH!

HEALING FROM PATRIARCHY'S CURSE OF TOO MUCH AND NOT ENOUGH

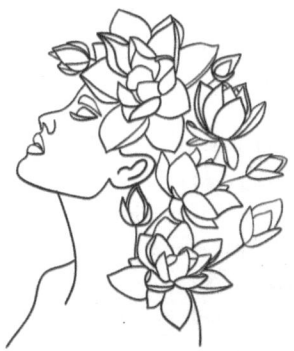

SARAH WHEELER

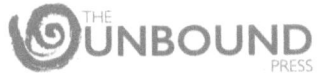

Copyright © 2023 by Sarah Wheeler

All rights reserved. No part of this publication may be reproduced, distributed or transmitted in any form or by any means without permission of the publisher, except in the case of brief quotations referencing the body of work and in accordance with copyright law.

The information given in this book should not be treated as a substitute for professional medical advice; always consult a medical practitioner. Any use of information in this book is at the reader's discretion and risk. Neither the author nor the publisher can be held responsible for any loss, claim or damage arising out of the use, or misuse, of the suggestions made, the failure to take medical advice or for any material on third party websites.

ISBN 978-1-916529-01-4 Paperback
ISBN 978-1-916529-02-1 Ebook

The Unbound Press
www.theunboundpress.com

Advance Praise for *Enough!*

Absolutely incredible read. From start to finish, I was hooked. It's written from the heart, as always with Sarah's books. It has stories from her past as well as dives deeper into the real reasons why the curse of too much and not enough is needed right now in our lives. I love that Sarah has researched history and has documented it in this book.

It's such a fantastic read and one that you can easily pick up and put down. The journaling prompts and meditations are great, and the words keep you in suspense as to what will be next. Sarah has gone through so much in her life and she isn't afraid to share it. This is a totally open book and one which will resonate with a lot of women.

Thank you so much for this incredible book. Sarah truly needed to write this to share with the world and it will certainly help you to be guided on your healing journey and beyond. I love the witchy parts in it as I can certainly resonate with that. Love love love it.

> Gemma Nice. Yoga Teacher, Relationship Coach and author of *BEE FIT, Baby Enhanced Exercise Fitness*

Wow, this is a powerful read. Buckle up for the ride! If you want to wake up and shake up your awareness of how you've been conditioned to feel not enough, and simultaneously too much, by patriarchy, history, education and the rest, then you need to read this book.

It boldly depicts feminism in a way that rings so true, but I couldn't have articulated it myself in the brilliant way that Sarah does. Easy to read, whilst uncompromising, Enough is an essential read for all women, and anyone who knows a woman!

> Claudine Nightingill-Rane, Body Image, Mindset and Blue Health Coach

A fresh take on patriarchy that really hits home how we, as women, have been conditioned to never feel good enough and never feel we do enough. With her signature and restful style, Sarah guides you away from the 'curse' of patriarchy's effects and towards a more compassionate and authentic way of being. A truly special book and a strong voice for women everywhere.

> Sameena Ali, Founder of Awaken the Goddess Festival.

Hey unbound one!

Welcome to this magical book brought to you by The Unbound Press.

At The Unbound Press we believe that when women write freely from the fullest expression of who they are, it can't help but activate a feeling of deep connection and transformation in others. When we come together, we become more and we're changing the world, one book at a time!

This book has been carefully crafted by both the contributors and publisher with the intention of inspiring you to move ever more deeply into who you truly are.

We hope that this book helps you to connect with your Unbound Self and that you feel called to pass it on to others who want to live a more fully expressed life.

With much love,
Nicola Humber

Founder of The Unbound Press
www.theunboundpress.com

Also by Sarah Wheeler

Shadow & Rose: A Soulful Guide for Women Recovering from Rape and Sexual Violence

2020 Vision: A Year Like No Other.
A collaborative book by authors of The Unbound Press

Access your *Enough!* content at
www.youreenoughyoga.com
with this code: **iamenough2023**

CONTENTS

Enough!	1
1. Beginnings	7
2. The Portal: Setting the Space for Your Journey	15
3. Founding Fathers – How Did We Get Here?	23
4. Remembering Our Witches	35
5. Enough Already: Owning the Alchemical Process of Recovery	43
6. Rest Is a Pathway Back Home	53
7. Allowing Imperfection	63
8. Busy Girls and Good Girls	83
9. Body	107
10. Blood	137
11. Fucking	153
12. To Mum or Not To Mum. That is the Question	181
13. Enoughness for Sale	195
14. It Is Not All in Your Head	207
15. Cult	227
16. Power	251
17. Nothing To Prove	281
Parting Words: Living as Enough	289
Recovery Resources	293
Notes	297
About the Author	301

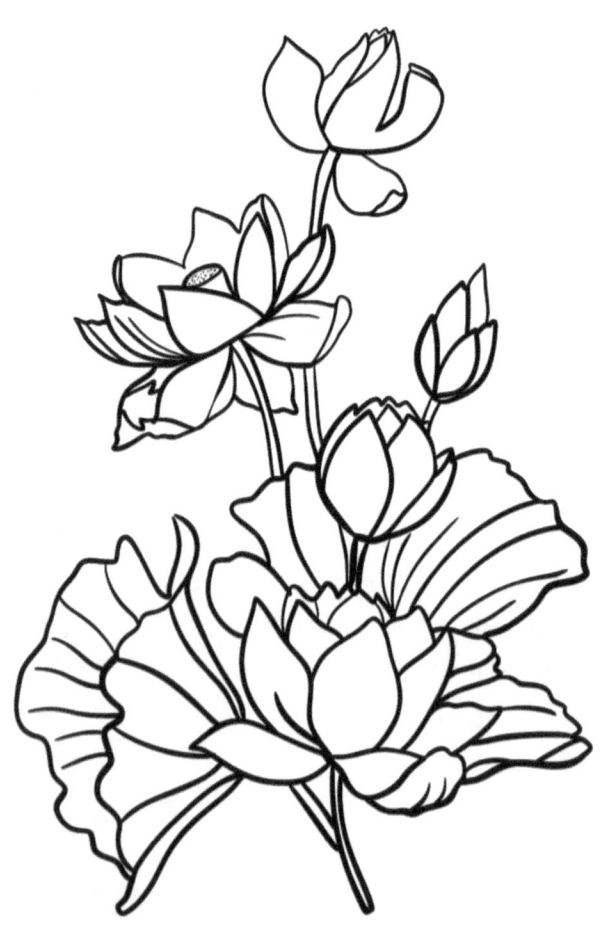

Enough!

On March 13th, 2021, patriarchy's curse of too much and not enough pervaded our screens and media. Women gathered in sisterhood circles to hold vigil for Sarah Everard. Murdered by an undercover Metropolitan Police officer, Sarah's body had been found mercilessly dumped in woodlands in Kent, England. Peaceful activism group Reclaim These Streets had jumped through every Covid-safety-related hoop to attempt to liaise with the Met to allow the scheduled gathering at Clapham Common, London, to go ahead. Feminine energy unfolding, hot footing its way through the toxic paradigm's red tape to be able to not only reclaim the streets, but to cling to the human right of gathering to protest, to mourn our dead. Red tape marked with women's blood. We wanted to create candlelit circles across the UK to remember Sarah, to be visible and heard as our hearts, tears, minds and mouths said:

Enough Now. Men, stop murdering us. Stop your bullshit entitlement that society taught you. Stop raping us. Stop touching us. Stop leering at us. Stop coercing us. Stop abusing us. Stop censoring us. We are not yours. We belong to ourselves. We are not here for you. Stop it all. Fuck patriarchy.

Reclaim tweeted in the afternoon of March 13th that having done the work to ensure safety at the proposed Clapham vigil, to satisfy the looming powers that be, the Met had failed to engage with their safety plans and suggestions. Reclaim's lawyers' interpretation of the law that Covid restrictions did not mean a blanket ban for all protests failed to make a difference, while a judge ruled that the High Court would not intervene to allow the peaceful vigil to go ahead.

The Old Boy's Club rode again. Patriarchy ruled that women gathering in face masks and socially distanced was too much of a risk while Covid was doing its thing, despite deaths and cases falling in the UK's lockdown 3.0. The message was clear. We were too much for society to allow us to be seen and these women had supposedly not done enough to ensure safety.

The collective Feminine intuition did not believe this had anything to do with Covid. How anybody failed to join the dots and see that the Met was trying to protect its own by standing by the murderous bastard Wayne Couzens, who stole Sarah, is beyond me. But then I am a woman and I am probably overreacting, being hysterical, seeing patterns that aren't there because I am too much and I don't know enough about the facts, right? Please.

Vigils went ahead in a number of other cities. In Bristol, women gathered, and each held a tiny flame to remember Sarah and every other woman killed by men. The police stayed back, they knew their place; *do not infiltrate our grief.*

The gaping holes in Sussex Police's so-called investigation into the death of Blessing Olusegun crept to the forefront at the vigil in Brighton. Why had I never heard of Blessing? Blessing was a Black woman found dead on the beach in Bexhill, East Sussex, her cause of death said to be drowning. Her family and friends do not buy it, and nor do the circles of women. On reading about this case, I remembered the racist murder of Stephen Lawrence and the Metropolitan Police's corruption in failing to fully investigate the men whom it was known in Eltham, Southeast London, had knifed Stephen to death. Will the truth be told one day? The truth that the police have failed Blessing as they failed Stephen?

The horrifying images we saw in the media of young women restrained in hog-tied submissive positions by male Met officers at Clapham Common will forever be a pox on London policing. Held down on their fronts with men standing over them. These women are every woman who has been physically and emotionally held down by a man. Abuse of women is effectively decriminalised in England due to prosecution and conviction rates remaining so low. These women are every woman who has been restrained by patriarchy because she is too much, because men are shit-scared of our power and will stop at nothing to make us believe that our supposed 'too much' is not enough to let us rise.

The Met's actions on March 13th depicted so devastatingly the patriarchal curse on women. This is the curse of too much and not enough. They acted out the curse by blindly following orders. They showed us that the system says: women in groups are too much, showing up is too much, our grief is too much, our outrage is too much, our rage is too much, our strength is too much, our persistence is too much, our tears and wailing are all too much for them. They try to impose on us the belief that we are not enough to be seen or heard or taken fucking seriously when we say that violence against women must end, because they are the system and they can do what they want. They try to show us that we are not enough to fight back but we are too much to be listened to. They act out the myth that women are not enough, not deserving of safety and a platform from which to be heard. They are not only found within the police. The patriarchy are the self-serving government, they are religion, they are the justice system, they are the benefits system, they are the powers that be which simply exist to spawn more tentacles of power because for patriarchy, no amount of power is ever enough.

Patriarchy is bullshit. We are enough. We are enough to warrant visibility, voice, representation, debate, law changes, health, money, an end to police brutality, the calling out of racism and misogyny. We warrant convictions for those who abuse power through corruption, and we warrant the seeking of justice against those who abuse us. We women warrant respect for our planet and for her bounty, which patriarchy attempts to bleed dry.

The curse of too much and not enough has infiltrated the story of women. Perhaps it *is* the story of women, our untangling, unravelling, breaking out from the binds of patriarchy. Our story is one of alchemy, of turning the lead of our oppression into golden sparks of rising.

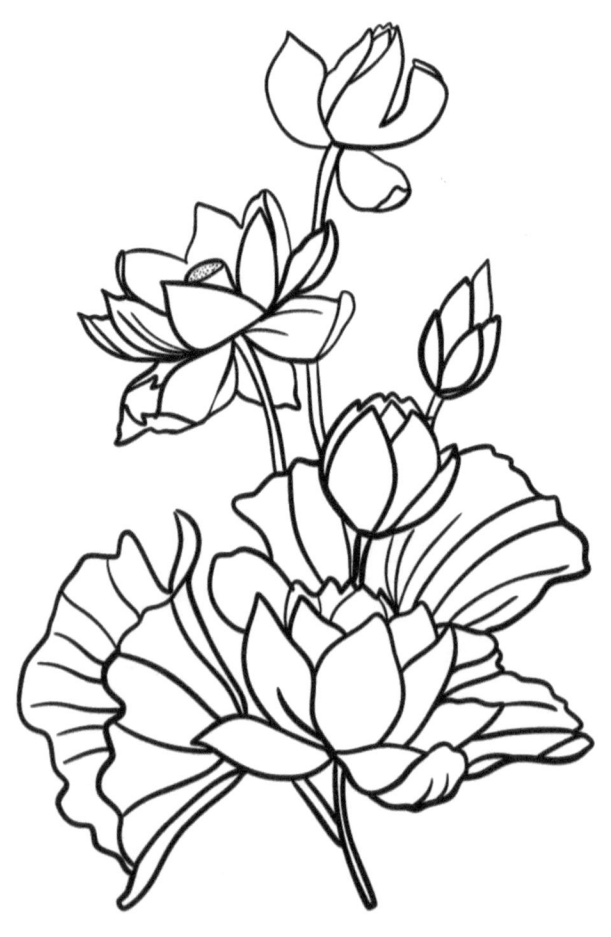

CHAPTER ONE

Beginnings

I'm offering you my hand, let us walk together.

Bring your 'I am too much'. Bring your 'I'm not enough'. Bring your fatigue, your messiness, your confusion, your brain fog, your rage, your self-doubt. Bring me your nice girl and your wild woman. Bring your wholeness, your magic, your glow, your genius. Lay it bare because it is welcome here. You are welcome here.

There is nothing you have to do to warrant being here, to know that you belong. There is nothing you need to do to make you deserving of the time you need to recover from the curse of too much and not enough. There are no conditions, no hoops to jump through, nothing to measure up to, nobody to compete with because this book is a space that is just for you.

I want women to be fully, openly, lustrously, and unrepentantly ourselves. I want to create spaces which nurture women's realisation that we are enough, just as we are. The pain of living with the belief that you are too much or not enough is pain that I wish women did not carry, but we do. Too much and not enough are within us, but do not belong to us. It is a curse we have lived with for aeons, born into us through the struggle, trauma, pain and conditioning of those who came before us.

The curse is a control system within the system which bows to the rich white male and attempts to belittle and marginalise those whom it decrees are less than. The system does not offer respect to those it does not recognise as resembling itself. Patriarchy breeds power and control through its tentacles of racism, classism, ableism, capitalism, and if you happen to be a woman, you can add misogyny to the intersections of these isms which may already be marginalising you. Patriarchy needs women to be run ragged under its curse to keep us out of the way.

If all of us women were well, rested, fully empowered within the knowledge and experience of being enough, then we would be fucking dangerous. Dangerous to the system that seeks to keep women oppressed through preoccupation with trying to have it all or get it all done, struggling to be the fullest expression of themselves while busily trying to make ends meet. The drive to have it all and get it all done was sold to us by patriarchy, packaged for us as the temptation of being Superwoman. Let me break it to you: you will never get it all done.

Women would be dangerous because we would be wise to the curse and its falsity. Instead, we would choose to nurture ourselves back into the truth of who we are. Back into our glory, our power, our magic, our goddamn enoughness, and lifting up other women while doing so. Healing ourselves little by little and being healed by seeing the women around us rise, stepping into their enoughness. We would reclaim and own the places we've already earned as change-makers across the platforms where we already show up and weave our magic; in board meetings, politics, arts, justice, parenthood, education, health and so many more. We would show up from the place of enoughness without anything to prove. We would no longer be competing with ourselves and each other to prove we could do it, to prove we could make it in the man's world.

Yet truly, those of us in the West have it easier than women who are fighting the curse under regimes like Iran and Saudi Arabia, where women battle to uncover their glowing enoughness while demanding the right to education, an income, healthcare and basic freedoms which we take for granted in the West. But I can't pretend that some of those struggles do not exist for the Western woman too, albeit in a less brutal form.

In the UK, we are not likely to be stoned to death for adultery, unlike our sisters in Saudi. In the UK, US, and Europe, we know women are unfairly paid for the work we do, whether it be in the boardroom or as home care assistants. We know we are marginalised by Western medicine and its lack of understanding of our cycles. We know we live in a rape culture where jokes about sexual violence are normalised on television. We know that when we speak out about these injustices, we are labelled as Feminazis or simply as uptight, too vocal, too much. We don't need to look at statistics to feel in our bodies and know in our hearts that this oppression is real. Patriarchy casts its shadow upon humanity, with women being fucked over most spectacularly in the male-favouring social milieu, where women must navigate the headfuck of a riddle that is the curse of too much and not enough.

If I had been given a pound for every time I was shamed by others or myself (most upsettingly) for being too much or not enough, I would probably still be writing this book but doing so from a penthouse or sprawling barn conversion in the English countryside. I believed I was too much when I cried for hours at a time as a teenager but struggled to explain what triggered my tears. The pain poured out of me while my heart felt so heavy it was surely going to drop through my body into the Earth and keep going before getting burned up in molten seething layers. Hot tears snaked down my cheeks while I berated myself for not being clever enough, pretty enough, thin enough, popular enough, achieving enough, driven enough, enough, just not being enough. The tears just came and came, my body would lurch and shake as I tried to find the words to express the pressure building inside of me; *whatever I do is not good enough. When I show my emotions, I get in trouble. I walk around ashamed and I feel trapped. This is fucked!* I felt like I couldn't breathe.

I was so used to living with the familiar pain of not enough that I unconsciously directed myself towards a career in which being rejected for not being good enough was part of the scenery. Yep, I was an actor and faced the constant barrage of competition, perfection-seeking and endemic levels of not-enoughness. I got out but the curse followed me.

The curse of too much and not enough was invented by patriarchy and the impact is real. Living on the swinging pendulum of worry that you are too much and/or not enough is damn stressful. In studies carried out by the Health and Safety Executive between 2010 and 2016, it was concluded that women are one and half times as likely to experience stress than men. The study cited factors such as the all too familiar work/life balance being a forerunner in the exacerbation of stress, as well as the prevalence of a 'do it all generation' of women who are somewhere between holding down a couple of jobs to put food on the table or pounding out a career, while also dealing with the unequal proportion of unpaid labour they take on at home including raising children and/or housework, emotional labour (emotional labour consists of making plans with one's partner, having all the extended family birthdays on the calendar plus sending cards and staying on top of the family's Google schedule), combined with unrelenting social pressures to be good looking, sexually attractive, a good friend and a general unattainable level of Wonder Woman standards. Dr Judith Morhing at London's priory clinic cites this untenable stress as being underpinned by 'living up to an imaginary Feminine ideal'.[1] I agree.

I am no psychiatrist, but I do hear anecdotes of these same pressures from women who attend my yoga classes and workshops and come to me utterly exhausted for Reiki treatments. Women have grown up believing we are not enough if we don't accomplish all this shit but we are too much for wanting all the good shit. Our whole being, body, mind, and soul swing between too much and not enough as we also slay it to compete with other women, as we prove we are enough because we have all the stuff like letters after our names (if you have had the privilege of a university education), a sweet little family, organic food on the table, money flowing in to pay for the OK house and the leaky kitchen roof, a wardrobe of clothes from Cos, hair dye to cover the greys and a thigh gap Angelina Jolie would be proud of. Once you have all that shit, the game is to prove you have it together emotionally and are not being too much by suppressing the tears, panic, exhaustion, stress and niggling aches at the adrenal glands. Let's not ignore the fallacy that we must not shine too brightly or be too successful lest we steal something from another woman who is also scrabbling around to be successful in the shadow of the curse.

Woah, that was a lot … go and make a tea if you need one. I felt frazzled just writing that paragraph!

What would life be like if you woke up every day knowing you are absolutely-no-doubt-so-fucking-enough? Daydream about it. Let yourself go there. What choices would you make? What would you let go of that drains your life while you try to compete to earn your space on the planet? We'll keep coming back to this as we journey together through these pages.

You can write your Enoughness Musings in this book if you like. I am a huge fan of annotating books with coloured pens, underling the words that resonate with pastel-shade highlighters, circling parts to remind myself to reflect on the bits that get me triggered or that I disagree with. I think this is because it was drummed into me as a child that it is wrong to write inside books, that they must be kept pristine … WELL, A) my female brain is a messy one, and B) I reflect best when I can jot down my responses in real-time upon the closest thing to me, whether it is the book or a napkin. So, feel free to go ahead and get the margins messy wherever you like on these pages because they are yours.

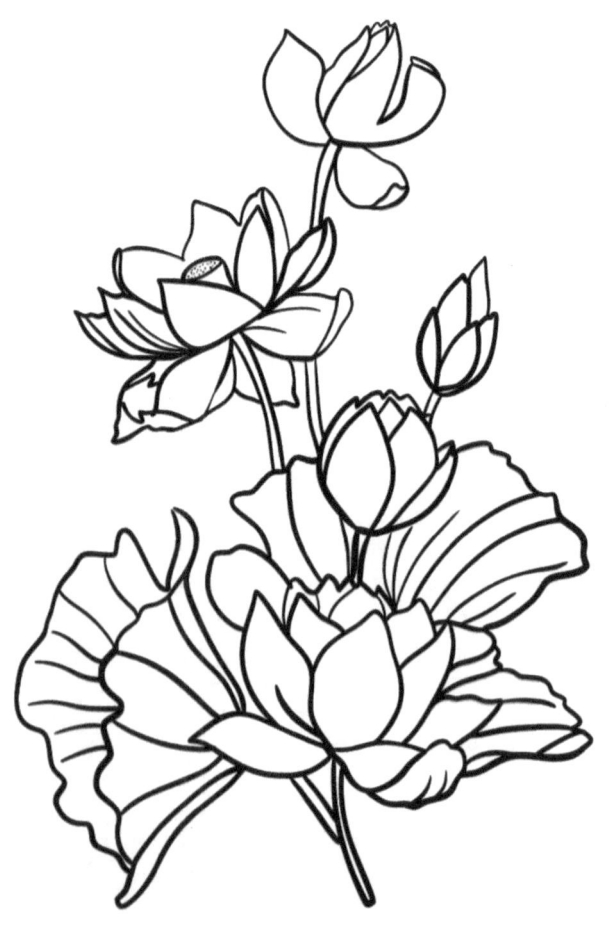

CHAPTER TWO

The Portal: Setting the Space for Your Journey

I don't believe that everything in our lives is pre-determined. I don't buy into the idea that every single obstacle we face in life is some kind of cosmic theatre performance which will have us act out the binds of karma from our previous lives, contrary to the teachings of much new age spirituality and the wellness industry which I work in. Some obstacles will help us to heal and grow, others will not. Plus, the adage 'what goes around comes around' is not always true. Some good people seem to always get dealt a shitty hand, and some nasty people seem to always come up smelling of very expensive roses.

I am a witch, though, and I do believe in past lives, and that past-life regression can help to shed some light on strong opinions, beliefs, or even unexplained body pains we may hold in this lifetime. Our past lives contain the age-old struggles of women feeling persecuted, controlled, being manipulated into believing they were too much or not enough or both. These struggles have also been bred into us through ancestral unresolved trauma from our Mother lines. What I do not believe is the premise that bad stuff we did in those past lives outright determines the hand we get dealt in this life. For example, I feel incensed when karma fans suggest that children born with disabilities are playing out some sort of penance for a transgression from a former life, that the child's soul chose to come and live in a body with catastrophic brain damage or incurable illness supposedly for their highest good, or the new age explanation for poverty: *I guess some people are just meant to be poor if they can't manifest their way out of it?* Tell that to the five year old who lives on a rubbish dump in South America. Somebody suggested to me once that the sexual violence I survived was part of my karma, something I 'needed' to experience for my soul's growth, pre-woven into my life's path. I wanted to punch them. Atrocities like abuse and terrorism are for nobody's highest good. To me, those ideas about a pre-determined life path are magical thinking and spiritual bypassing of three-dimensional problems such as unfair distribution of wealth, misogyny, age-old corruption, racism, colonialism, inequalities based on socio-economic factors – all of which stem from patriarchy. Let's also not forget that randomly sometimes bad things happen to good people, and annoyingly, the world's psychopaths, sociopaths, and narcissists get success served to them on a shiny silver plate. Urgh, those fuckers.

I do believe though that life presents us with portals. If you remember the TV series *Stargate SG1*, you might have seen huge circular portals open to take the crew through the cosmos when they use their portal-opening device. Well, I have zero evidence to show you about those portals being real (soz), even though I love the idea of stumbling across a shimmering, luminescent gateway to another dimension where you might even meet yourself in a parallel universe! I believe that there are moments of our lives when we might feel aware of consciously choosing a path, of going this way or that when given the opportunity to pause and take a new direction. These moments are portals. Think Alice in the Tulgey Wood in her Wonderland, faced with many signs pointing up, down, back, forward, this way or that. Alice doesn't know what path to take and concludes with the help of the Cheshire Cat that it doesn't matter which path if she does not know where she is heading. The difference is that you do know where you are heading because you have had enough. Enough of the people pleasing, enough of the shape-shifting, enough defensiveness, enough confusion, enough competition, enough making it, enough Superwoman, enough world's best mum/wife/sister/daughter. You may not know what the path will look like, but you can feel the pull toward a new place where people live free from patriarchy's curse. When you picked up this book, you opened a portal, a hidden threshold was crossed toward a world where women are recovering from the patriarchal wounding so ingrained in womankind. This book and your choice to open this portal reflect the gradual rising of the Feminine energy they try so hard to control, maim, silence and exterminate. I want you to know that I am right by your side with my words in a sisterly way as you journey through these pages and into the practices.

We are going on a journey of remembering, reclaiming, revisioning, recalibrating, revitalising. It is a journey far deeper and more timeless than the scope of this book. Enoughness is a journey of Feminine energy. Your Feminine is your wisdom, your ancestry, your heritage, your creativity, your light and your darkness, your badass wild witchy warrior queen who resides in your heart and belly. Enoughness is a journey through body, mind, and soul to meeting your highest self, your spark of creative life force who can strike light and life out of the fresh, nothingness of the void. Reclaiming our enoughness is remembering that there was a glimmer of ourselves that existed long before we had a name. She is the spark that glowed before your body came here and will exist long after your body is buried or burned to ash.

Chapters 7-17 of this book are curated around three themes: Rest, Recovery and Rising.

Rest: I'm going to explore the importance of rest for connecting with one's inner enoughness a little later in this beginning portion of the book. But for now, consider that postponing rest until after your work is done is a symptom of patriarchal control. That is why I am placing a rest or Yoga Nidrā practice at the opening of every chapter so you may bring rest as a priority into the forefront of your life, or at least while you enjoy this book.

Recovery: This will be the chunkiest piece of each chapter where I share stories with you based on my own recovery from the curse of too much and not enough. I hope that my insights, stories, and the voices of some other people that I have woven into the book will shed light on the wounds that patriarchy's curse may have caused other women. Recovery is finding the pieces of ourselves which got lost or harmed, pouring care on those wounds and considering how you may coax out change in your life to empower the whole, absolutely enough person that you are.

Rising: In these pieces, you will find invitations for gentle actions to help align you with your enoughness, actions that can help shed the curse of too much and not enough. I will share with you nuggets of breathing practices, journal questions for reflection, and artistic ideas.

Before we go any further, I want to acknowledge that 'being enough' might mean different things for different women. Whatever 'enough' is for you, I want you to know that I am SO here for that, to excitedly cheerlead or gently encourage the blossoming of your own expression of enoughness while you are held in the energy of this book. It is absolutely cool if, at this stage, you are unsure of what 'enough' means for you. Life has a rather anti-Feminine habit of requiring us to problem solve, react quickly with a level head and give coherent responses even when, at certain times of our cycles, we may feel the opposite of coherent.

Amongst these pages is not a place where you will be rushed, and there is certainly no need for right answers when it comes to untangling from the curse of too much and not enough. And by 'right answers', I mean the socially acceptable ones which we give to reinforce the myriad hats we end up donning, for example: the nice girl hat, the intelligent hat, the rational hat, the good mother hat, the good partner hat. How's about you put on your 'let me be real' hat?

Let's have a little practice now, if you want, to explore what enoughness means for you. You will need:

- some paper (use this next page if you like)
- a pen (or several coloured pens)
- a candle
- some gentle music (I like to listen to DJ Taz Rashid, MC Yogi, or Stars of the Lid for some heart-shifting, chilled-out vibes)

Light your candle. Take a seat or lie down nice and comfy. Place your hands on your tummy, and take some easeful, slow, soft breaths through your nose, so soft that there is no noise from your breath. Repeat this breath pattern for a few rounds until you are feeling softer and settled. Play your music in the background and take a rest before picking up your pen. Ask yourself the question: *What would enoughness feel like?* When you intuitively feel it, you can make notes, write prose, doodle, or mind-map your response on the next page. Enjoy.

What would enoughness feel like?

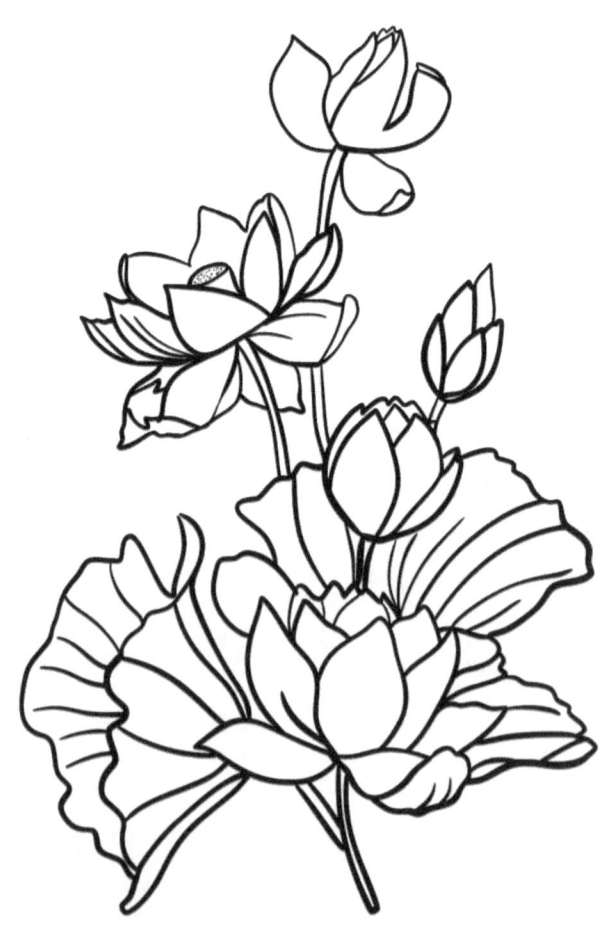

CHAPTER THREE

Founding Fathers — How Did We Get Here?

If She was already here, always knowing that we are enough, how did we forget our enoughness? I don't think there was one specific moment when a bunch of old, bearded, Feminine-fearing men held a board meeting at Patriarchy HQ and decreed from here into eternity:

> *let it be known that women are cursed to lives of exhaustion, competition and struggle. To live disconnected from their wisdom, blood and bodies so that we men can dominate the Earth's narrative and marginalise anybody whom we do not recognise as part of our Old Boys' Club. We will endeavour to create a narrative which suppresses women's health, voices, and bodies, meaning they must shape-shift into perfectionism in order to find a male to mate with so our planet can stay populated. We will celebrate when the boy children are born and mourn the arrival of girls. We hereby declare that women must not be unruly, angry, decisive, rich, empowered, autono-*

mous, aware of their magical healing abilities, promiscuous with anybody other than their designated male, allowed to gather with more than one woman at a time (we don't want them cooking up plans together and realising their collective power), for this will simply be too much! We must cajole them into being polite, sweet-natured caregivers and homemakers, ones who will never rock the boat or upset the apple cart, ones who will look after the whole family while staying on top of their ever-changing moods, ones who suppress their creeping doubts and the sense that something is wrong. They must never enjoy sex or pleasure but be willing to be fucked whenever we feel like it, they will learn to pretend to enjoy choking on our penises while they gag and their eyes water. Whatever we do, we mustn't let them touch their clitoris!!! If they fail at any of the above, they must believe that they are not enough and are completely replaceable.

Now, this does sound pretty convincing, but I'm sure the birth of the curse of too much and not enough did not go down this way. I believe patriarchy's demonisation of women and propagandising of the pro-male narrative began slowly and insidiously. The demonisation of women lives on in Christian cults who live the doctrine that women must live 'under their husbands' or 'under their fathers'.[1] The founding fathers of patriarchy played the long game to ensure the longevity of its insidious poisons – misogyny, racism, homophobia, and the over emphasis capitalism – which continue to blight humanity.

If we are to trace the origin of the curse of too much and not enough, we must look back into pre-Christian history and mythology, where we will hear stories of Lilith. Lilith is the original version of a badass woman who knew she was enough. Marcia Starck and Gynne Stern explain in their book *The Dark Goddess* that Lilith was not portrayed as a Goddess in early writings about her powers.[2] Lilith was depicted as a demon and seductress, even as a vampire, within a text called *The Sumerian Kings List*, dating back to approximately 2400 BC. Myths about Lilith from Sumerian, Babylonian, and Hebrew traditions emphasise her wildness, her connection with nature and wild beasts, and, most pertinently, her sexuality and refusal to submit to any authority. Lilith's unfavourable reputation within early patriarchy stems from her sex life as Adam's wife (yep, Creation Myth Adam from the Bible's Old Testament) and her unshakable will to be her own boss, advocate for her own body and desire. The story from the Jewish Talmud features Lilith's major transgression of refusing to lie underneath Adam during sex.

Like a true Feminist, Lilith questioned why she should lie beneath Adam. I believe that Lilith wanted a debate about why they couldn't mix things up in their marital bed and what this meant about their positions (pardon the pun) in their relationship. Clearly, this Lilith's desire for sexual pleasure and healthy debate were too much for Adam and the old-school Jewish scholars writing the Talmud. Adam wasn't having any of it and decreed that he must take the superior position in sex and in their whole relationship.

According to Starck and Stern, 'Lilith uttered the name of God and flew off to the Red Sea'. In Hebrew lore, the Red Sea is a shady place where demons hang out. Unsurprisingly, this is where the writers of these myths decided she must stay because only a devil woman would dare to assert her right to equality with her husband. I'm not surprised that Lilith flapped her wings to flit away. I don't blame her.

Lilith is completely excluded from the Hebrew Creation myth in the Bible's Genesis. Her story is marginalised into absence. Her behaviour, which we can interpret as being a badass, sexual, Feminine force of nature and totally enough without her male partner, didn't make for exemplary reading for the target audience circa 1200 BC. I used to go to Sunday school as a child until about age seven. I would hear stories from the Old Testament about how God supposedly created a man first (naturally, the Old Testament's patriarchal writers would say this because men were seen as SO much more important than women) and secondly made the first woman out of one of Adam's ribs (WTF?). This woman was Eve. For Christians, the story goes that Eve screwed things up for humanity because she got tempted by the Devil in his snake costume and chose to bite an apple from the Tree of Knowledge. Eve's disobedience and thirst for wisdom was a big no-no, so God banished Adam and Eve from the Garden of Eden. Not only were they cast out because Eve wanted too much (to be more than just her husband's wife), but God decreed that women must suffer atrocious pain in childbirth thanks to Eve. I did not quit Sunday school because of the fantasy stories about creation but because of the number of rules, the obsession with obedience, and the unsatisfactory responses when anybody questioned the stories. *Can we prove God is real, and if he is real, why does so much bad stuff happen?* The teachers would answer: *because it says so in the Bible.* I remember thinking, *Why is God a man, why not a woman?*, but I never dared to ask my questions. I just remember thinking that the people who wrote the Bible, whomever they were, seemed to have a problem with women because the females in the Bible were portrayed as up to no good, for example, the insistence that Mary Magdalene was simply a prostitute rather than a teacher alongside Jesus. (Incidentally, there is nothing wrong with fully consensual, non-trafficked sex work.) *They must have thought girls were bad,* said my seven-year-old wisdom.

There is disagreement between the scribes of the Old Testament and the authors of the thirteenth-century Hebrew Kabbalah as to the origins of woman. Kabbalists were mystics of Judaism, and this movement became popular in the Middle Ages, while the Kabbalistic book of the 'Zohar' brought a mystical slant to the Old Testament.[3] In the Zohar, we find Lilith described as being made from the shell that surrounds the moon and as being the original epitome of Feminine energy. She is separate from Eve and Adam but her influence is felt in Eve, who wants to express her Feminine energy, which is so suppressed and punished within the writings of the Old Testament. My interpretation of the Lilith stories is that patriarchy painted her as both too much and not enough. Too much for wanting equality between husband and wife through discussion of the sexual needs and desires of women, too much for even venturing to ask her questions of Adam, and too much for refusing to acquiesce to Adam's (and patriarchy's) insistence that she just get beneath her husband and shut up. They wanted to make an example of Eve too, after she and Adam ate an apple from the Tree of Knowledge of Good and Evil. The anti-woman Old Testament authors wrote in Genesis chapter three, verse sixteen: 'To the woman he said, "I will make your pains in childbearing very severe; with painful labour you will give birth to children. Your desire will be for your husband, and he will rule over you."' Well, that's that, then. Thanks, patriarchy!

The writers of the first half of the Bible wanted women to know they deserved pain as punishment. Worldwide, women are shamed simply for being women, as if having a vagina is a source of shame, and the ultimate agony of the searing pains of childbirth are our just desserts for supposedly fucking up in Eden. I believe that having a vagina, or better yet...wait for it...a *cunt* is a bloody excellent privilege because it is the opening to the pulsating power source of the root and sacral energy centres. To me, cunt is not a curse word. It is just too much for patriarchy, like the name of Goddess Kunti from The Mahabharata, one of the epic Sanskrit texts. Goddess Kunti, exalted as a mighty female, embodies the power of the female body, the beauty of the vagina (yoni in Sanskrit), modelling for us that being a woman is not a reason to carry shame. Shame does not belong to women – it has been projected onto us by patriarchal religion and culture.

Old Testament writers wanted women to know that they must be ruled by their husbands because they cannot be trusted to resist temptation. They wanted women to know that we are not enough without a man to watch over us, and too much for wanting a taste of wisdom from the apple. Without a man to live under and lay under, what might women get up to? Some modern Christian sects, such as the Fundamentalist Latter-Day Saints, continue to shame women for being women through these outdated beliefs, indoctrinating them with the myth that they will be out of control without the husbands, fathers, brothers, and pastors. Patriarchy wanted to protect itself from Feminine power by keeping a close, coercive watch over women. Pain is what they say we deserve, physical pain and the emotional pain of living inside patriarchy's curse. We have had enough of making the emotional pain invisible. We have had enough of too much and not enough.

Woman and Man Stuff

Patriarchy has not only fucked over women, but men too. I know that may be hard to believe, but please humour me! Before we go any further into this rabbit hole, I want to be super honest. For me, it seems as if the scourge of believing we are not enough is predominantly a pain felt by women, and I believe the message of believing in one's enoughness is more pertinent to women than men. Why? Because society is set up to show men that they are supposedly more important than women with its gender pay gaps, lesser representation in female Members of

Parliament, and endemic levels of domestic and sexual violence against women which never gets prosecuted. Society teaches men that they are held in higher regard than women, with more room to manoeuvre.

BUT it would be remiss not to notice that patriarchy causes problems for both women and men. Patriarchy has styled its own versions of what it means to be female and male, plus it can barely wrap its narrow-minded head around what it thinks of people who break gender stereotypes. Patriarchy wants to control women because they believe us to be overly emotional and out of control, so they cajole us to stay ignorant of our power and keep a smile on our faces. On the flipside, patriarchy compels boys to be boys: hard men, out of touch with their emotions and concerned with order and logic. The system has no time for traits which it considers Feminine, or in other words, illogical, irrational or 'just too much'. Yet both men and women are encouraged to disconnect from themselves at the emotional level. Showing and honouring emotions has been labelled for men as 'woman stuff' or 'gay' in the derogatory sense, therefore out of bounds for men because emotions have become synonymous with what it is to be a woman. For women, expressing emotions in the form of anger or tears is called 'overreacting', but it seems slightly more palatable for society to see a woman cry than a man.

Men have emotions and they bloody need to feel them, allow them, and speak about them. Every man I have dated, including the spiritual and polyamorous chaps, has told me they struggle to talk about their emotions:

'We just didn't talk about that stuff in my family. My dad never said much about that. We just got on with things.'

I've heard this line so many times.

'I do sort of want to say how I feel. I don't know how, though. Then I get embarrassed for not knowing how and embarrassed for feeling embarrassed.'

It breaks my heart that men want to talk about their emotions, fears, traumas, dare I say it, shed a few tears, but society has made it a no-go. I wince whenever I hear parents invalidating and gaslighting their crying children by saying to them, *Stop being silly*. Strangely, I feel it more deeply for the little boys because when little girls get a bit older, they will get together and form networks for anything from gossip to blubbing that they got dumped. Who do boys blub to when they need to let it all out? It is not because men are fundamentally bad at dealing with emotions, particularly those of their female partners, that we do not see men speak freely about what is on their minds. I believe it is because society has labelled women as the 'emotional ones', and so men have been conditioned to be reluctant to go there. If more men were talking to each other, checking in about the stresses in their lives, there would be less male suicide. Allowing men to feel their emotions and speak about them takes more than a pint and watching the football with the lads, even though this is a good start. We need men to start saying:

'What's been going on for you? / I have been feeling X about X lately, how about you? / I've not seen much of you recently, you OK, want to catch up?'

If you have been affected by suicide and would like support, do check out the resource list at the back of this book.

Basically, patriarchy wants women to smile, keep a lid on it and stop being too much, so it can protect itself from the huge revolution ushering in the collapse of white male power (I promise you, it is coming). Patriarchy needs men to stay anything from stoic to totally emotionally unavailable in order for the worldwide System to continue treating anyone who is not a white, heterosexual male so abominably. If enough men started to feel their own emotions, their pain, empathy on the planet would increase, and then whole swathes of men may consider the pain of others, different races, different age groups, their ancestors, partners, wives, daughters, mothers and grandmothers. If parents teach their sons to unashamedly feel their feelings, speak their feelings and enquire as to the emotions of others, the suffering of all people under patriarchy would decrease.

Gag Us, Bind Us, Burn Us. Watch Us.

Black Lake Reflect Us, Cleanse Us,
Hold Us, Rebirth Us.

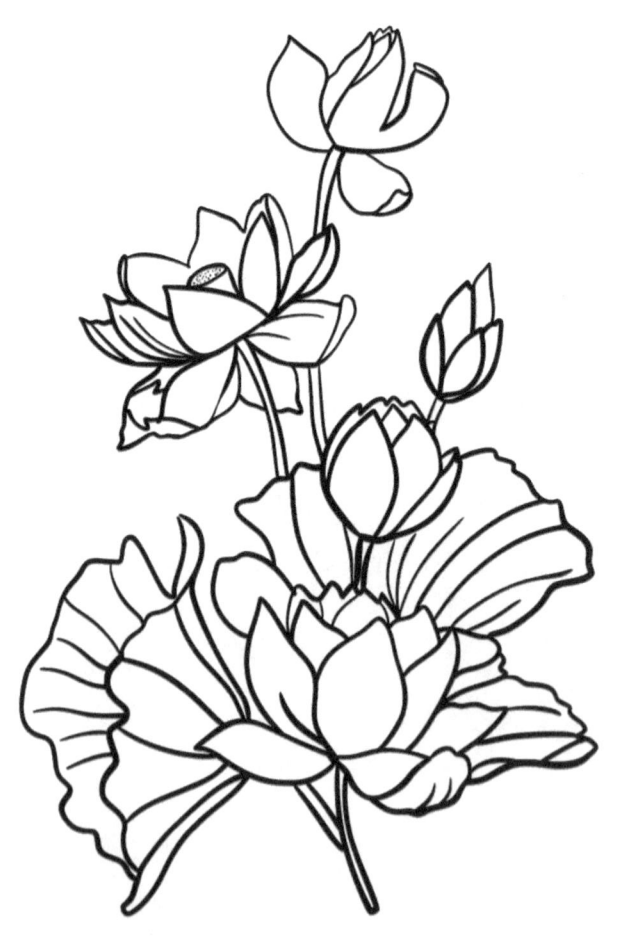

CHAPTER FOUR

Remembering Our Witches

The curse of too much and not enough was in its heyday while rampaging through Europe from around 1400 until the early 1800s. I heard about the European witch hunts and trials briefly in school, but nobody named it as genocide. The rough estimate is that sixty thousand people across Europe were murdered by execution after being tried for witchcraft. Around three-quarters of those murdered were women, which makes the witch hunts a gendercide.

Women were systematically hunted due to a fervent belief propagated by the upper echelons of the Christian Church that some evil, chaotic force was out to overthrow Christianity in its populist forms of Catholicism and Protestantism. Remember the bad rep cast onto women thanks to the myths of Lilith and Eve who dared to question the word of their man and God? What a perfect way to turn man against woman and women against women by making pious Christians believe that women were going to be the cause of the downfall of religious order. The unsavoury reputation of women was reinforced by a text called the *Malleus Maleficarum* which served as a manual for how to spot a witch and how to interrogate her. According to research on control and totalitarianism, the *Malleus Maleficarum* was the first handbook on brainwashing and coercion to fulfil an end goal, which in this case was the extermination of wayward people who were a supposed threat to the Church.[1] The witch-catching manual echoed the sentiment of Old Testament writers: women deserved all the pain, suffering, banishments and servitude to atone for Eve's supposed transgression as she boldly and rightly took a bite from the Tree of Wisdom: *Of course, women are the threat to religion and order*, said the 16th-century patriarchy.

History shows us that not all witches killed in the genocide were women, but the vast majority of women murdered on the premise of saving Christianity points to the systematic purging of Femininity from the planet. They wanted everyone to believe that women were more likely to be witches because of the Church's perception of us as untrustworthy and uncontrollable, thanks to Eve's taste for the apple. They wanted Feminine energy gone, tortured, raped, hanged, burned, stoned, broken, drowned, aborted, wiped out. They wanted what was decreed in the Bible: 'Let woman learn in silence with all subjugation ... Adam was not deceived, but the woman being deceived was in the transgression' (1 Tim. 2:11-14). Women were framed as the destroyers of humanity's innocence by Old Testament writers. This defamation was used again as the false reasoning behind the Reformation of the Christian Church after the gendercide. They persecuted us because of our mighty transformational power that exists in the vessels of our bodies, because of our wombs, our inner cauldrons where we carry out our alchemy. They cast us as malformed and evil because we bleed, because we possess the power and portal to carry and birth children, to sense that wisdom is available for all, not just for those with a penis or those called God. They burned us because they were scared of us, and Europe's population bought it. Not surprising, given the amount of anti-woman sentiment in the Bible, which those old-school God-fearing Christians lapped up. Seriously, if you can stomach it, search online to find anti-woman statements in the Bible and you will find some shockers. It was written in what reads like a grotesque biblical prophecy, 'Thou shalt not suffer a witch to live' (Exodus 22:18). They burned us because they said we were too much to live with but not enough when compared with the men. All men were Adam and all women were Lilith/Eve.

I am very sure that I am descended from witches. I have no historical evidence to base that on ... yet I will never forget the burning desire I had to enter the Witchcraft Museum in Boscastle, Cornwall, aged about five, and the hot tears of grief I shed when told I was not allowed. Aged 17, it was like a homecoming when I crossed the threshold into that cold, dank museum. I experienced that familiar sense of home once again when I took part in a shamanic journey held by Priestess Rachel Smithbone with my writing circle.

Rachel guided us through primordial sound and meditation to the Black Lake, where my former wise woman sisters stood in community, waiting for me. Pieces of my soul were returned to me during the journey. Pieces that were wounded long ago by the curse of too much and not enough. Witches were the wise women, the seers, healers, midwives, herbalists, oracles and fortune tellers of yesteryear.

I asked Rachel about the importance for women of connecting with our witchy ancestry. She explains:

Whether we actively identify as witches or not, connecting to our inner witch is about connecting to our innate Feminine power. As women, we have been systematically robbed of this power, robbed over lifetimes, robbed over generations. There is a deeply internalised, implicit understanding that this power is unsafe. What we now see so clearly is that our Feminine power was never unsafe for us – but unsafe for a distorted and destructive patriarchal order. The time has come to step fully into the power of our inner witch. We are ready to shed generations of ancestral trauma related to Feminine wisdom, energy and spirituality. In this integration process, we will reclaim the wisdom and leadership that stalks angrily in this repressed archetypal shadow and in doing so, start to rebalance the external power structures.

Remembering the witch is an important aspect of the journey back to wholeness. The witch is both an archetypal energy and an ancestral energy within us all. The cost of female persecution, especially on the grounds of spirituality and power, has struck a damaging blow to the psyche of all women. This inner remembering of the witches is especially potent for women who have explicit memories of this past life persecution. The 'witch wound' keeps us bound in trauma – in the suppression of our power, we also suppress our unique soul gifts. The witch wound keeps us separated from our sisters and in deep fear of stepping up and speaking out. In short, it keeps us trapped in fear.

Thank you, Rachel, for your badass insights!

Any woman who feels a connection with nature has a connection to the witches; whether you like to run barefoot into the woods, paint your nails black, occasionally hug a tree, let out a gut-wrenching howl or enjoy the scent of dew on the grass or whether you dab your menstrual blood onto your body as a blessing (yes, I am that woman), an echo of the witches lives within you. All of these acts could be labelled as too much or over the top, or some could say there's not enough evidence to prove the healing power of these acts. I disagree and reclaim these acts as essential to the reclaiming of the sacred Feminine energy from the system which shamed Her and us. As much as I write this book for you and me, I write this book in honour of the witches and all those killed for beliefs that will never fit the patriarchal mould.

Enter The Void With Me.

For There Is So Much To See In The Dark.

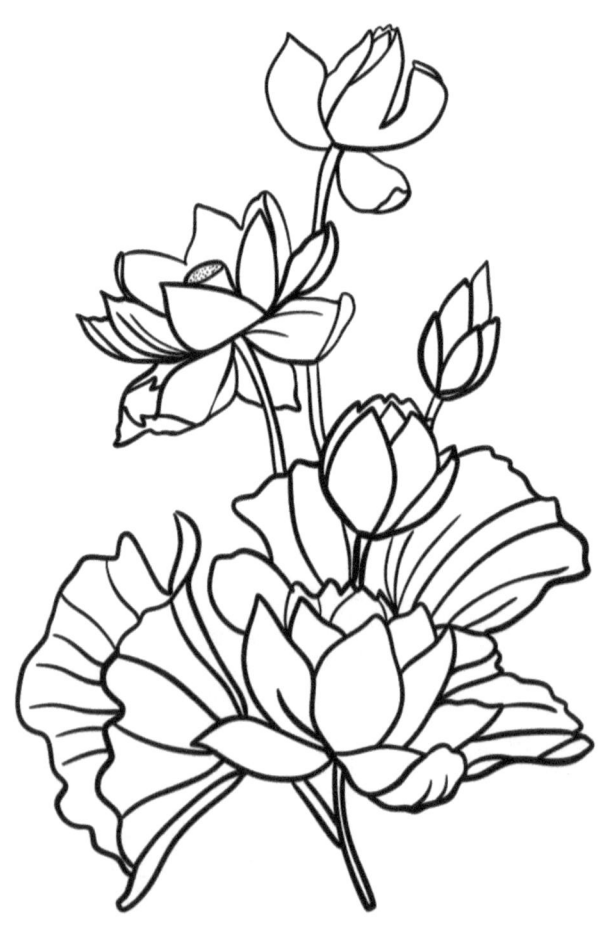

CHAPTER FIVE

Enough Already: Owning the Alchemical Process of Recovery

You are doing something magical by even beginning to consider that you are enough. I invite you to consider yourself an alchemist while reading this book and exploring the meditations and journaling. Think of Mickey Mouse in the film *Fantasia*, conducting a chorus of dancing broomsticks while he accidentally coaxes out the power of the sorcerer's hat. If you haven't seen it, take a few minutes to enjoy that bit of the film on YouTube. Alchemists delve into a process that in medieval times was considered more than science; it was magick.

Alchemy is a process of transmutation, which is the action of changing one thing into another or catalysing a state change into a different form. Traditionally, alchemy focused on either turning lead into gold or concocting an elixir to promote eternal youth. Let me break it down for you before we go further: you are already precious, like gold, and you are the keeper of the elixir. While you lovingly sift through and witness the beliefs and patriarchal conditioning that tricked you into believing you are too much and/or not enough, you are encouraging a state change to occur by revealing the precious gold of who you are. This change has the potential to unbind you from unhelpful, limiting, or unkind ideas of yourself. When we habitually believe the thoughts we think about ourselves, we are inadvertently growing a thorny, endless maze in mind and body where our true enoughness is trapped.

I had a book of fairy tales and nursery rhymes that lived at my grandparent's house. I loved to cosy up on my nan's sofa and hear tales of princesses, beanstalks, and golden geese. Let me tell you a fairy-tale now. If you are sitting comfortably, I will begin. A beautiful Maiden is trapped and exhausted, tramping around the unforgiving terrain of the thorny maze day after day. The maze lies deep in the dark forest, where surely she will not be found. Her feet bleed. She tends her wounds only for the cuts to split open again and again as she walks the labyrinth, the paths turning her around and around, curling back on herself. There is no way out. Our Maiden yearns to get free, to be rescued. Enter the drop-dead gorgeous prince astride his trusty steed. He hears her sobbing and spies blood seeping onto the leafy path from her lacerated feet. He draws his sword and slashes open the maze, revealing the woman picking thorns from her feet. He scoops her into his embrace. Quick as a flash, she is freed, leaving the treacherous maze in their wake. They fall in love instantly and ride off into the sunset. *Hooray!* the reader yelps, *She is saved, all she needed was the man to free her from the maze's spiky torment.*

Except it was not the man she needed to set her free, it was herself. Even Feminists like me love a love story, and there is nothing wrong with finding a partner to share life with. The problem is that our Maiden in the story is still trapped by her belief that she is not enough to save herself. Perhaps we could retell the story like this. Swap the prince for the woman's identical twin. The twin has ventured into the deep dark forest to find her sister, lost to her so many years ago. She always believed she would find her sibling, the other half of herself. She would find her no matter what it took. She hears her twin's sobbing and spies blood seeping onto the leafy path before her. She has no weapon to sever the vines, but she knows she must find a way inside the maze. She calls to her despairing sister: 'It's OK, my love. I am coming for you.' She loops the long, heavy sleeves of her dress over her hands, and although her fingers are restricted, she works the vines to untwine them. Time passes and she keeps untwining. Some of the vines are knotted tighter than others, with more thorns and thicker foliage, but still she works, prising the branches apart to create an opening. She spots her sister, and they embrace. Tears flow. 'I thought nobody was coming', sobbed the Maiden.

'No, my love,' replied her sister. 'I was always coming for you, but these things take time. It took me a long time to find the deep dark forest, and longer to pick my way through to you. Some of the vines are stuck fast, we will need to climb our way back out.'

'We can unpick the knots together,' said the Maiden. 'There is no rush now we have found each other.'

The identical twins worked on the twisted vines for three days and three nights. Their fingers and feet bled. They nursed each other's wounds. Finally, they made an opening deep enough and wide enough to bring them out to the edge of the maze. Hand in hand, the sisters stepped through their portal together. The Maiden looked out at the open fields surrounding her, ready to reclaim her life.

The lost twin needed the mirror image of herself, her identical twin, to save her. To remind her that she was not lost forever and was able to untangle her way back to freedom. Together, the women unravel themselves from the maze which kept the Maiden trapped for so long, out of touch with the unshakable part of herself that knew she could get free. The vines are her beliefs which kept her ensconced in not enough, resigned that the maze was too much and would keep her walking its paths, feet bloodied forever. Perhaps this is a familiar tale? Two sides returned to one another, just like the myth of Goddess Inanna, who rescues her twin sister Ereshkigal so that their ancestral pain can heal.

Sometimes the thorny maze may appear to be endless, but we needn't spend endless time out of our lives unpicking the vines. Yes, there is no need to rush, but it is helpful to acknowledge our progress on the path to enoughness and to discern when the inner work you have done is indeed enough work. There is a trope within the personal development/professional development/healing/spiritual communities that purports there is always another layer to peel away, another level to complete, another promotion to prep for, always another piece of karma to clear while people are undertaking a quest for betterment, clarity, or as one spiritual organisation promotes, the task of 'polishing our lives' so that we can 'shine with wisdom'.[1] Trust me – you already have wisdom whether you have polished yourself or not. This trope, left unquestioned, may leave people searching, navel-gazing, chasing tails forever and forgetting to acknowledge progress and enjoy their remembered enoughness. Alchemising the unhelpful beliefs stored by mind and body, which may hold us back from claiming our enoughness, certainly is a process of unfolding. Imagine an opulent swirling rose which seems to be infinite when we look into its centre. But healing work can turn patriarchal when it feels like there is endless work to do, another task to tick off the dreaded to-do list so that we can measure up and 'shine'. Who gets to say whether we are shining or not anyway? The invisible judge of shininess? Women are feeling creatures. We know when we feel repelled by something, when something is not for us on a particular day, be it sitting in a board meeting, minding our friend's children or attending a self-development seminar; some days, we just do not feel like doing that shit. I assure you that it is your prerogative to listen to your feelings, heart, and gut if you feel you have done enough alchemy to reclaim your enoughness.

One of my favourite pieces of yoga wisdom comes from the *Yamas*, which are a set of ideas for how to conduct ourselves in life. Trust me, I like to be a rule breaker and dash away dogmatic ideas, but this one is so supportive when allowing ourselves to reveal our inner enoughness. *Santosha* is the idea that we can allow ourselves to be contented with our efforts, to be satisfied and autonomous, to trust that we have done enough or had enough. Trust yourself on this journey. Alchemising the inner wounds which have led us to believe we are not enough or too much is an autonomous journey that I hope unveils your sense of when to say, *Yes, I'm ready for more,* and when to say, *Nah, I will come back to this later* (and later might be months away!), or most crucially, *Nope I think I am good where I am, I feel content with what I have done, and it was enough.*

Discerning when you are content or enough may go against the grain of patriarchal conditioning of pushing through, getting one's head down, sucking it up and seeing something through to the end, even when it does not feel good or the timing is just a bit off. This way of being is way more suited to males because it correlates with and reinforces their daily rhythm, which is governed by the circadian rhythm. Go, go, go, work hard, play hard, grind out a result each day, the day peaks when a result is produced, followed by rest for the same pattern to continue like clockwork the very next day. To me, 'circadian' sounds like the name of a Roman emperor – pretty appropriate because we know that the Romans loved a bit of patriarchy (thanks a bunch, Emperor Constantine). Women are not governed by the circadian rhythm, although it is very much believed that everybody should be vibing to the beat of this male-favouring rhythm. We have another inner clock called the infradian rhythm that allows us to feel more cyclical. The infradian rhythm is what spins our monthly cycles, whether we still bleed or not. It's not helpful to listen to the mini, invisible emperor sitting on our shoulders telling us we need to dig in, get on with shit and finish it by the end of the day. For example, reading new information and learning may come easily one day, whereas perhaps the following week, we want to throw the book at the wall because we cannot concentrate, and we would rather be down the pub with a friend, enjoying some yoga, or binge-watching Netflix. In the same way, rooting through, witnessing, and holding ourselves in self-compassion as we discover we have been living bound by patriarchal conditioning may not feel like an appealing prospect every single day because, like I said, the process can feel heavy as you look at parts of your inner emotional landscape that you have disowned. I invite you to pick up this book when it FEELS right and good or like you need a dollop of sisterly love, not because you started it so you must finish it! I invite you to read when you will be less likely to be disturbed. Make yourself a warm drink and snuggle under a blanket each time you pick up this book. We are here to recover from and alchemise the myths of too much and not enough. Alchemy was never rushed.

Western society's male-dominated system coerces us to be in a forward-facing go-mode all the time. I don't know about you, but I have found this exhausting, and I don't even have any kiddos to look after. The coercion is the ingrained belief that our families, jobs, fitness regime, social credibility (yes, in China, there are Social Credit systems that one must stay on top of. FYI, the system says playing video games is bad and being a parent is good, and if journalists write about the credit system, they will no longer 'qualify' to travel or own property[2]) and financial welfare will all cave in if we dare to down tools, stop the action and rest. I used to catastrophise this belief that life cannot function without me, as well as desperately aching to say, 'Stop the world I want to get off!' I would sit spinning in my office chair at 8.30 am before my colleagues had turned up, rocking it from side to side, bouncing between fantasies of slinging my coat on and legging it from that office, never to return, or feeling paralysed by an insidious fear that if I got off the metaphorical hamster wheel, life would collapse around my ears. Would I let my colleagues down? Would I be broke and homeless within a couple of months? It is so easy to fall into the crevasse of believing that there is no time to stop and take stock, to literally take a time-out of the marching pattern of being useful and productive, to check in with one's inner voice and see what she has to say underneath all the plate-spinning and keeping-the-shit-together façade. Rest is resistance to patriarchy's endless productivity.

There are millions of women around the world who are the sole providers, single parents living on the poverty line or way below it who will not have the same level of privilege that would enable them to flounce out of a job and risk having no income for a few weeks to take a rest.

This inequality and injustice are the work of patriarchy which affords men the opportunity to leave women with their children to raise with only minimal legal recourse and financial support. It is simply not fair that some women (mainly rich white women) have the opportunity to easily leave the binds of gruelling jobs should they wish to, while many women in marginalised groups are unable to make this leap at all or with any speed, due to the prevalence of socio-economic inequality. Those of you reading this book, I am guessing, have the socio-economic privileges to be able to designate some time for real rest, to literally do nothing. The reality is that taking sacred time out to restore and nourish oneself is not a possibility for every woman worldwide, but it should be. It is my hope and gentle request that if you are reading this book and can find your way to putting time aside to nourish yourself and begin to recover your beautiful enoughness, that part of your practice has a positive impact on the women who have not been afforded the same privilege as you, if you indeed see that you have been privileged. You may not have been privileged due to all those tentacles of patriarchy, but if you have, remember that and take action for sisters who do not walk in similar shoes to your own.

Here is a caveat: I do strongly invite you to use the resting practices woven into each chapter every day. Sure, you might not want or have time for thirty minutes of dedicated rest to embed into your daily schedule, but you will have time for ten, or even five. If there is no time for five minutes of rest at some point in your day, please make time. You can thank me later.

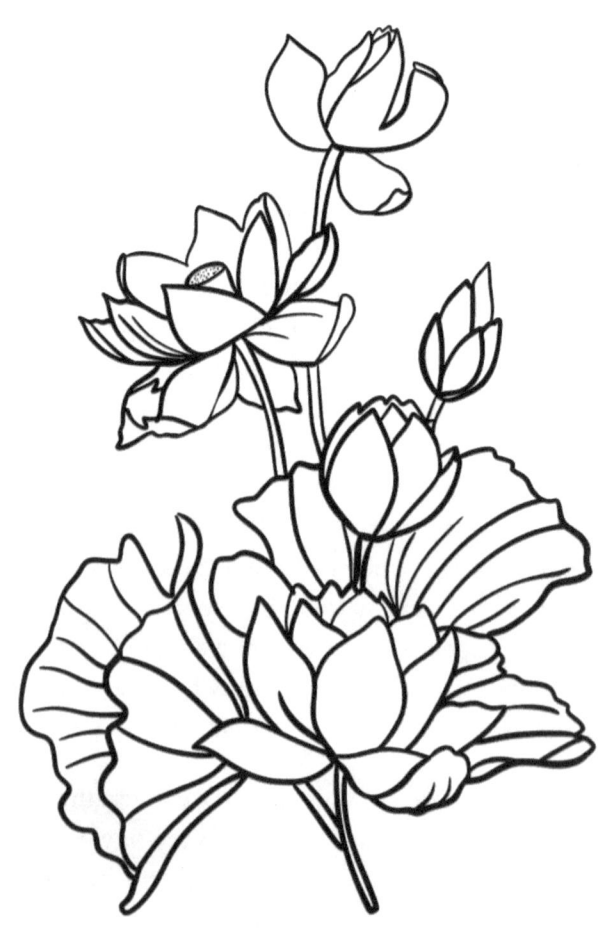

CHAPTER SIX

Rest Is a Pathway Back Home

It is easy and understandable to feel swamped by the enormity of the patriarchy monster. Left unchecked and unchallenged, the system will continue to reside within our relationships with ourselves, our loved ones, family systems, workplaces, education system, health, bodies, economy, justice system, policing, and medical establishments, to name just a few places where patriarchy makes itself at home, often unquestioned and left to perpetuate its own power while playing havoc with women's sense of enoughness. Making a conscious choice to rest (not in front of Netflix but with sacred, uninterrupted time) may begin to work its magic by letting the inner voice of wisdom come through so you can become aware of the subtle and not-so-subtle influence of patriarchy's favourite tropes: too much and not enough.

You will discover that throughout this book, I will invite you to try the resting practice of Yoga Nidrā. The cool thing about Yoga Nidrā is that it is a triple header of yumminess; it is a practice to explore rest, a technique for deepening rest, and the manifestation of the Goddess Yoganidrā. Yep, you read that correctly! Yoga Nidrā is a different kind of sleep. A space beyond the states of waking, dreaming, and sleep, where the body and mind rest while consciousness remains awake. Taking time and space for rest is an essential aspect of taking care of ourselves and each other. Regular rest in deep relaxation or Yoga Nidrā can help relieve stress and support healthy nervous system responses, which can alleviate the sympathetic nervous system from being 'stuck' in high alert. When the sympathetic nervous system is rather too active, people may struggle to be still, be bothered by anxiety and feel unable to relax into rest. Regular rest can help to 'calm and connect' with body and mind, a welcome relief from overactive 'fight or flight 'reactions. The impulse for fight or flight is appropriate when the body needs to evade an unexpected threat, but not so helpful for us if the adrenaline released by these protection reactions becomes the backdrop for daily life. Living under patriarchy can feel anything from mildly irritating to debilitatingly anxiety-inducing. The more that we can coax body and mind into rest while letting our awareness remain calm yet awake, we give the nervous system an opportunity to recalibrate and restore the inner sense of fullness, otherwise known as enoughness.

I would bet money on the assertion that the more a person experiences deep rest, the level of clarity as to what needs to be let go of from life will increase. In other words, we can discover what we have had enough of.

As a yoga teacher, I like to play with the idea of *Atman*, which was woven into yogic philosophy from Hinduism. *Atman* is a Sanskrit word that means 'the inner self or spirit'. Throughout life, we build up layers of personality, defence mechanisms, beliefs, and coping strategies, along with ancestral pain inherited from the lineage we are born into. Some beliefs and strategies are helpful for our success or survival, others are not. A belief of mine is: *I am too much because I am an emotional kind of person, so it is best to try to suppress how I really feel to keep myself palatable for others.* Generally, this belief and coping strategy would work for a while until my nervous system would get overtaxed, trying to keep up the appearance of looking like I always had my shit together. I would bottle up important things like tears and so-called negative emotions (also known as 'low-vibration' emotions within the spiritual community) because when I was a child, I concluded that people get annoyed by tears. We all have our own versions of these beliefs and behaviours, which our egos concoct to keep us safe from real or perceived threats such as social ostracization or abandonment. Our ingrained beliefs and behaviours get layered on top of Atman. Atman remains, but we have less chance of hearing our own true voice of wisdom because Atman is squashed under our beliefs that are all too often influenced by the curse of too much and/or not enough.

Rest gives the thinking and logical parts of the brain, which reside in the frontal cortexes, a much-needed break from its myriad tasks, which include behaviour regulation and self-control. Simultaneously, resting the body also signals to the older parts of our brain that they need not alert the autonomic nervous system for an episode of fight, flight or freeze. These three Fs are to be reserved for when we need to make a quick getaway, defend ourselves, or for when the nervous system perceives that it would be safer for us to freeze and do nothing rather than try to fight or flee. It is the sympathetic nervous system (SNS), part of the autonomic nervous system, which generates these appropriate and lifesaving reactions, especially if a person finds themselves under extreme duress, danger, or trauma-inducing events. Thankfully, humans have evolved to keep these essential functions because the three Fs are needed for survival. However, the SNS can get 'stuck' in activation mode, resulting in a person feeling edgy, anxious, nervous and sometimes struggling to navigate interpersonal relationships because the brain may be both scanning for danger and misinterpreting difficult yet harmless situations as real cause for fight, flight or freeze.

The 'stuckness' of the SNS is often a result of trauma triggered in a one-off event such as a traffic accident, an act of physical or psychological violence, a hate crime, hospitalisation during Covid, or an unexpected end of a relationship including grief from a break-up and/or bereavement. Over a couple of months, the overly alert state of the taxed nervous system may begin to ease as the person takes care of themselves by resting and seeking professional help to cope with what they have endured. Unfortunately, some people find that the anxiety, jumpiness and intense SNS arousal stick around for longer than the expected couple of months after the trauma-inducing event and may signal that this person is suffering from post-traumatic stress disorder (PTSD). Sadly many people have lived through more than one traumatic event, for example, survivors of childhood abuse (sexual, physical, emotional, or all three), survivors of domestic abuse, survivors of narcissistic abuse, refugees, war veterans, survivors of racial abuse resulting in race-based stress and trauma, and survivors of gender-based violence. Traumatised survivors of these scenarios may find themselves living with symptoms similar to PTSD symptoms which may include and are not limited to: body pain, anxiety, irritable bowel syndrome, flashbacks, emotional flashbacks, nightmares, hormonal imbalances, chronic stress, panic attacks, and difficulty sustaining interpersonal relationships.[1] If these symptoms occur over a number of years, it could be indicative of C-PTSD (Complex PTSD). The world is an unjust place and too many people bear the brunt of these injustices through marginalisation and trauma. Many of these injustices are correlated with living in a patriarchal system, for example, male-perpetrated violence against women and the scourge of sexual violence, with an estimated 20% of women being sexually assaulted since age sixteen.[2] I am one of these women.

Whether or not you recognise you are living with trauma, PTSD, C-PTSD or a general weariness with life, you deserve to receive compassionate, patient, professional medical intervention to help with what you may be experiencing. Learning to rest can complement professional interventions as a way to heal and undo individual wounds. Saying yes to rest is saying no to the system of oppression that keeps people too busy to take real time to nourish themselves. Perhaps you sense that your weariness or trauma may be linked with a lifetime of being acclimatised to surviving a system that does not honour difference nor the sacred Feminine and sacred Masculine aspects of yourself. Perhaps you are angry and exhausted about constantly adjusting yourself to avoid being too much or compensating for not being enough. I promise you that resting will help you remember who you are and that who you are is enough.

None of what I have written about the challenges around rest may apply to you. This may be because you have inherited a level of socio-economic privilege which meant you have not faced poverty or you do not have to work, therefore giving you more time to rest than most. I don't know that for sure, only you will be able to recognise any unearned privileges you hold should you choose to explore the matter. The point is that everybody's body and mind will benefit from real relaxation. Yep, even those elites who run the world (unless they are the narcissistic or psychopathic ones) would benefit from stillness, quiet, neither asleep nor awake in the liminal space watched over by Goddess Yoganidrā, should she grace one with her presence! They might hear what their real self has to say, the part of them that recognises the truth that their own liberation is intricately interconnected with everybody else's, including those whom they oppress and harm. Pressing pause on daily tasks and routines to take rest, or even better, replacing some of the to-do list that may gradually reveal itself as extraneous, in favour of pockets of slow movement or rest is a gentle practice of self-enquiry to explore how both too much and/or not enough came to be and the impact of patriarchy's curse upon your life. Maybe this all sounds rather doom and gloom? Let's be hopeful, though, because people, communities, smaller strands of the system are taking a new shape, messily finding the way in the dark to different ways of relating. Ways which honour difference, respect, autonomy, and freedom along with the values and traits of the sacred Feminine and sacred Masculine, no longer dancing to patriarchy's tune.

Living under patriarchy is tiring for so many reasons. Women around the world face and fight injustice and marginalisation from those in power, while living with patriarchy's unspoken yet visceral maxim that we are too much but will never be enough. The curse of too much and not enough lies in wait in our exterior and interior worlds, making the possibility of a frazzled nervous system a very real one. While we are tired, we find ourselves in a race, chasing an invisible prize which, once achieved, can only be satiated for fleeting moments. A prize so rarely won, yet the competition for it can be compulsive. I have been unwell because of the pursuit of this prize, have wasted hours of my life comparing myself with people both in real life, in magazines and on screen, and this was when I was growing up in the early 2000s while The Facebook was still a glimmer in Mr Zuckerberg's eye. The pressure for women to attain and maintain the prize of perfection can feel all-encompassing. I have a sinking feeling that for generations younger than myself, the exhausting, obsessive quest for the perfection prize is getting worse.

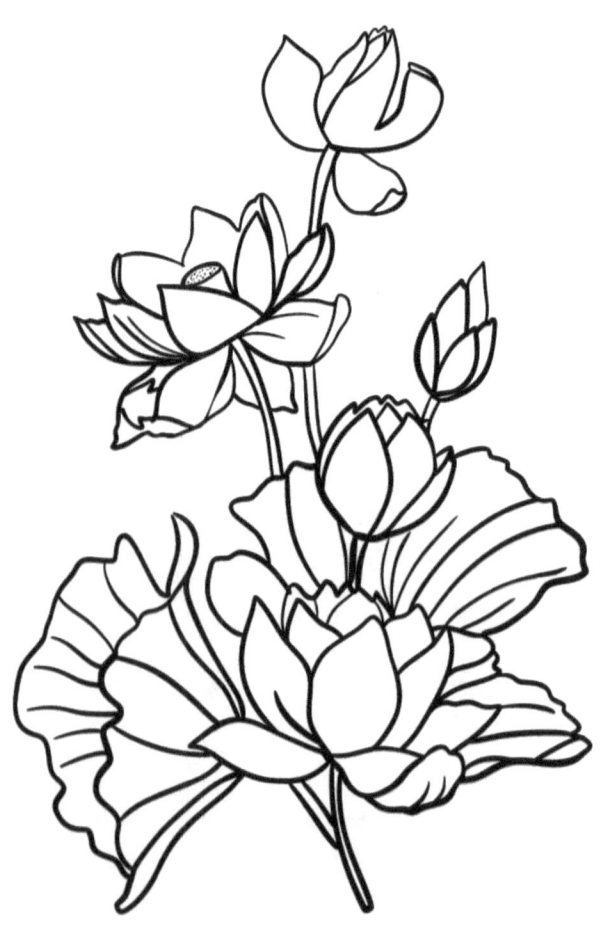

CHAPTER SEVEN

Allowing Imperfection

Rest

Before anything else, take a rest. Gather your comfy things like pillows and blankets and make a cosy nest for yourself for this chapter's Yoga Nidrā practice. Go to the *Enough!* area at www.youreenoughyoga.com and enter the password: iamenough2023

Recovery

> 'There's the pressure to be perfect all the time.
> The perfect picture, the perfect place…'
> – *Screened Out* documentary

When we are duped by the curse of too much and not enough, part of the psyche, in this case, the ego, tries to keep us safe by protecting us from the consequences of being judged as under par from society's expectations. Striving for perfection can become a bind which keeps us stricken, doing more damage rather than fulfilling the ego plan of keeping us safe. Researcher and Academic Brené Brown perfectly sums up the human drive for perfectionism: 'Perfectionism is a 20-ton shield we lug around thinking it will protect us, when in fact it is preventing us from taking flight.'

Humans used to live in tribal groups. Being accepted by the tribe was a matter of survival. Not so easy to survive alone thousands of years ago with sabre-toothed tigers roaming around as it was within the relative safety of a group. We are wired with a desire to belong and this desire remains, although modern living fiercely promotes the values of individualism, being the best and standing out from the crowd in the glory of being perfect. These days people want it both ways: to be accepted, validated by our groups, which keeps us socially safe, not outcast and vulnerable, while also trying to stand out within our social groups as 'the perfect one'. Even within our friendships, families, and workplaces, the pressure to out-perfect each other exists. With the explosion of social media, people build their individual brands on Instagram while living their #bestlife, enjoying the #perfectsunday and planning the #perfectwedding, all while deploying the right amount of wholesome sass to influence their followers. The pressure for women to appear perfect in all aspects of life is nerve-janglingly unbearable, but I am not pretending that other genders do not experience the pressure for online perfection too. If you have used any social media and you are not made of stone, you will have been influenced by the glossy lives and personal branding. Coach Carol Cavalante speaks to this aversion that humans have against anything which is less than perfect:

'We only want to make space for the good stuff, but it is actually the harder, more negative things that happen in our lives that we can take the biggest lessons from and at the end of it, understand ourselves better.'

Everybody's mind is vulnerable to idealised images of perfect bodies and perfect brunches as the background to pretty typography. Pre- Instagram, early humans learned skills which would keep them alive: tracking prey, distinguishing which berries and plants were safe to eat and, of course, the essential skill of making fire. It was a matter of life or death to hone these skills to avoid being served up for the sabre-toothed tiger's tea. In modern Western life, there are still reasons to hone skills, and without people perfecting their skills, we would not have lifesaving medicine, human rights lawyers, or bomb disposal experts. I am very glad that people in those professions have continued to hone their skills! Let's be real, though, it is not a matter of life or death if an exam is failed, a presentation goes to shit, a promotion is missed, social events fail to meet expectations, or the perfect eyeliner flick has not been achieved for posting online – except in patriarchal society, which hammers home the curse of too much and not enough. The pressure to succeed in daily life can be an emotional minefield.

Unfortunately, exam failures, presentations going tits up, imperfect social occasions, being passed over for promotion, and struggling to get one's make-up selfie perfect can feel like a matter of sheer survival. I don't care if that sounds too dramatic. There is something about being a woman that means something extra is demanded from us, that women must compensate for living on a sliding scale which labels us as too much or not enough.

Perfect versus Replaceable

When I was growing up, rooting around in the dark for what it means to be a human woman, I always believed that there would be a woman who was better than me, more deserving of life, so I must be the best version of myself no matter what. Life seemed to reinforce this belief. I had a Saturday job in a café when I was fifteen. I enjoyed chatting with customers, serving people what I used to call 'posh coffees'. The owners chose Motown, funk, and disco for the stereo, which added to the fun but laid-back vibe of this busy café placed in the high-end area called The Prom in Cheltenham. On the outside, I was a confident teenager but inside, the voices of not good enough played on a loop in my mind. My café job helped me to feel that I was something, that I was useful and I belonged. I used to people-watch the shiny twenty- and thirty-something women who poked at salads and sipped skinny cappuccinos. I presumed these women definitely had their lives together and were mega successful. I hoped to be like them when I reached my twenties. Looking back,

I am pretty sure these women did not have their lives together because who really does in their twenties, and who gets to say what a 'together' life looks like anyway? One Saturday, one of the other waitresses came in to start her shift, she was a couple of minutes late and in her rush to tie her apron on, did not say her usually breezy hello to the owners as she arrived. The couple that ran the café were pretty jolly when it came to chatting up the customers but did not think twice about publicly berating their staff. 'You need to sort yourself out and start turning up on time, and don't just ignore me and Garry when you arrive,' barked one of the owners to the late waitress. 'I've got girls queueing up to work here, you know!'

The owner shamed the late waitress loudly enough for staff and customers to hear. In her opinion, her girls, which was what she called us as if we belonged to her, were lucky to be serving coffee in her establishment and we were a commodity, easily replaceable at her whim. It was both warning and life advice for the young girls working there, which for me translated to: fix up, show you are worthy because there are plenty more where you came from. This moment imprinted my body and mind with an unquestionable belief that there is always somebody on the periphery, just out of reach but as if I can feel them, who is better than me because I am not enough. On reflection and through working with my patient therapist, I know that so much of my life has been lived in fear of imperfection and rejection, silently terrified of falling under par of what I perceived life expected from me. Perfectionism is a by-product of patriarchy's curse, inexorably tied to the myths that women are too much and/or not enough. Being perfect becomes a way to cheat the system and avoid being revealed as an apparent fraud who is not worthy of the career, job, success, partner, family, love, time, attention, or space on the planet. The nasty truth is that striving for perfection is the system. It is the continued effort to prove that we are OK, well-behaved, enough, worthy of inclusion and acceptance, unlike Eve and Lilith, ostracised for stepping out of role, too much for their partners but not enough to deserve respect or equality.

I think I would be remiss not to say that there is zero wrong with having huge dreams of a perfect life, being an alpha woman, ambitious, goal-focused and working hard to achieve one's dreams and then giving oneself a huge pat on the back for pulling off something brilliant. What is of interest to me is the felt experience of the driving force behind these goals; is it a nourishing or draining one? How about the possibility of exploring life by setting your own standards, not following the notions of perfection which are peddled to us by all kinds of media 24/7? If being perfect lights you up, even just some of the time, then crack on and keep chasing perfect. It might be helpful to explore whether your goals are fed by striving to prove you are enough and live up to perfection. What if women chased their dreams from a baseline level of enoughness, knowing we are enough without the outer trappings of Instagrammable perfection? I am finding that I feel increasingly fulfilled, stable and healthy when I do not share images that paint a picture-perfect version of myself (or any images for that matter). Plus, the 'Gram is already saturated with images of white yoga teachers, so I think the world will cope without seeing tons of images of yours truly. Humans are not built for endless perusing of social media feeds or the bombardment of fleeting moments of false perfection. I do not want to fuel the social media cycle which predominantly only shows the best bits of life, the 'perfect bits'.

Body Perfect = Picture Perfect

In case you had not noticed, I am massively unsettled by the perfection myth, which is beyond endemic across social media. I feel this because I want to protect the vulnerable pieces of me which are still healing from many years of an eating disorder. It is crucial not to overlook the damage that images of perfection can do to people who have eating disorders and conditions such as body dysmorphic disorder (BDD). Eating disorders do not always manifest themselves by driving a person to get very thin, as is symptomatic of anorexia nervosa, but these disorders generally arise from the sufferer's belief that they are not good enough, flawed, not acceptable and that their life is not within their control. What feels controllable is food intake (and sometimes exercise) and this disordered relationship to eating becomes the exterior manifestation of an inner, secret emotional pain. My disease was anorexia and I believe it is truly patriarchy's disease because it wants to keep the sufferer small, constrained, oppressed and fragile. I never wanted to be fragile, I wanted to be perfect, but anorexia had a plan which left me weak and ill. I wanted to be the best and to show it with my body like a badge of honour, to be the one who has it together, the thin one. I remember feeling like everybody else was allowed to be who they wanted to be, weigh whatever, eat whatever, but the disease will not allow its host these same rights. My mind was not my own under the disease. Eating disorders are like parasites which take over the body, mind, and all of life by running the same thoughts, same beliefs, same rituals, same habits, same restrictions every freakin' day.

Even now, every so often, a voice in my head that tells me I would be a better person if I was thinner, if only I could reduce myself down even smaller from a size 8 to a 6, and then a 6 to a 4, and then what? A mortuary slab? Anorexia does not care, it is the disease that keeps on giving you hell until you have nothing left. It will cheat you into trying to be perfect while killing you in the process. Unfortunately for those friends and family members who have to watch the sufferer shrinking away, reasoning with anorexia does not work. Solace can come from uncovering the painful beliefs, often attached to interpretations of life events, which triggered the need to restrict one's intake of energy from foods that keep us alive. Anorexia wants to destroy life force, but any physicist will tell you that energy cannot be destroyed, it only changes form. The life force which anorexia attempts to steal can be restored by getting help to witness, understand and heal the pain under the outer symptoms of control, restrictions, and fasting.

These days I am able to notice when I am having thoughts about food restriction. I thank my brain for sharing its repetitive narrative, and then I consider what these old thoughts may be a reaction to. Perhaps I feel stressed, unsafe, anxious, ineffectual or like I am losing control because I am not #livingmybestlife compared with any random person that my brain has chosen to fixate on. Perhaps fear of abandonment has been triggered because my partner remarked about a female colleague being really nice (wow, my little upset self gets very freaked out by that one!). I hear and witness my thoughts and try to give them space. Yoga and meditation have been game changers when it comes to no longer getting sucked into downward thought spirals as I get to breathe, and the thoughts have space to breathe and dissipate. After breathing, I can comfort myself, remembering that I do not need to act on destructive thoughts about calorie restriction or judgemental thoughts that berate me for not being perfect in the ways that patriarchy wants. I'm not going to lie, though, it is really fucking hard. Comforting myself might look like letting out tears, drinking herbal tea, taking a walk in fresh air, or just telling a trusted somebody how I feel. (Trusted somebodies are people who will let you talk without trying to fix, find solutions or coach you about how you feel without your consent. Leave therapy to the professionals!)

On one of my writing breaks to the beach, I felt shaky and upset because I judged my body as old and fat compared to the bodies of other women at the beach. I know these thoughts and slight panicky sensations well enough to know that acting on them will not have good outcomes for me. These thoughts have been indoctrinated by the patriarchy machine which teaches girls and women that body fat in supposed wrong areas is not desirable. If a woman has some flab, she is not a perfect specimen. It is more socially acceptable for a bloke to have a beer belly than for a woman to dare to show off her body at the beach if she is less than a size ten. Instead of beating up on myself for yet again having anorexia thoughts, I placed my feet on the warm pebbles, both hands on my heart and let a few tears roll down my face. This attack of not good enough began to pass as I allowed myself to feel what I was feeling with a little dose of self-compassion. When I was in the grip of the disease, I would have upped my exercise and calorie-restricting if I experienced an episode of feeling less than perfect, remaining prisoner to the eating disorder's loop of unhelpful thoughts coupled with destructive behaviour.

Perfectionism abounds. If I were a young person today, I know I would not be coping well. I am so damn glad that smartphones were not a thing when I was growing up. How can we calm the inner voices that trigger the drive to be perfect when we have a device in our hand that offers both distraction and connection while enticing us into apps which push people toward perfectionism? Firstly, nobody is immune to the Instagram perfection parade when one spends a lot of time on social media being bombarded with aspirational images. The algorithms of social media serve us with tons more content on the endless scroll than our brains, eyes, and nervous system can cope with. Too much scrolling is now recognised as eliciting the same physiological responses found in motion sickness: heaviness, fatigue, dizziness and nausea.[1]

It is no wonder that Steve Jobs, former CEO of Apple, would not give his children access to iPads before he died in 2012. Tech does not serve us content because it cares and wants to help. The industry's algorithms obviously do not care about our wellbeing, but they will give you more of what you spend time looking at so that profit can be made from the user's attention. If you look at fluffy animals, then more cute critters are brought to your feed, but if you follow celeb influencers who have supplements, make-up, diets, and gymwear to sell, guess what you see more of? All while more money flows to overly paid celebrities who profit off paid posting. I recently unsubscribed from a popular spiritfluencer (spiritual influencer) after I noticed she had an affiliate link to a rehydration product she was touting while decked out in her tiny pastel-coloured coordinated athleisure wear. Her whole blog post was there to promote the product, which looked embarrassingly obvious. Sure, there is nothing wrong at all with monetising one's work – as a freelancer, I know that bringing in the cash is essential – but it would be good if celebrity influencers would stay in their lane.

I know that my mental health suffers when I visit Instagram more than twice per week. It drags out behaviour from me similar to how my teen self behaved when I devoured too many images of models in tween mags, and later frequent readings of *Heat* and *Grazia*. The less opportunity I give the influencers, the better I feel. I hate to be a party pooper, but you may benefit from a social media detox (the only kind of detox I enjoy these days!) if you feel like your mind is getting scrambled and wellbeing suffering from too much scrolling. You do not need to go cold turkey, perhaps you might put your phone away in the evenings, leave it in another room while you hang out with your children or choose to take an undistracted phone-less walk for 20 minutes per day.

From Fixation to Meditation

Meditation may also help with unhooking from the influences which drive perfectionism. You do not have to be good at meditating or sit for hours on end to reap the benefits. Ten minutes of quiet time, keeping the mind gently focused on the breath, will begin to bring some relief from a busy mind of unhelpful thoughts. I began meditating nearly ten years ago thanks to the nudge toward mindfulness meditation from my GP, Dr Jo, who I am sure was sent to me as divine intervention. She was the doctor who diagnosed me as having anorexia and body dysmorphia. She was very clear that anorexia is a disease which I could recover from, it would be hard, but managing my state of mind would be part of my recovery. 'Don't expect miracles from this,' she said, 'but it will help.' I struggled with the practice for a couple of weeks. *Fuck this, I can't stop thinking! My thoughts about how shit I am get even louder when I try to meditate.* The meditation app

I used told me that this was all part of it, that mindfulness is not a technique to stop thoughts, yet over time the practitioner would grow accustomed to witnessing their thoughts and allowing them to pass by. In my case, this meant no longer hooking on to my brain's chatter about not being good enough, followed by spiralling down into destructive behaviour like starvation or self-harm.

Mindfulness continues to be part of my ED recovery, my detangling from perfectionism, and my ongoing healing from the patriarchy's curse of too much and not enough. Building my practice of meditation and mindful breathing has helped create enough space for my mind to experience a window of opportunity to respond when I feel hijacked by the perfectionism pattern. Years after my appointments with Dr Jo, I still have shitty thoughts about myself and occasionally get jealous and insecure that I no longer have the body of a sixteen-year-old, but a steady and consistent meditation practice has radically shifted how I respond to those thoughts. It feels like mental freedom that I never thought I would have. If you recognise you have a consistent inner monologue which berates you for a perceived lack of perfection about anything and everything, and this monologue drives you toward behaviours that cause you physical or emotional harm, do yourself a favour and consider finding some therapeutic help. I have listed some resources at the back of this book.

This Book is Not Perfect

While writing this book, I have had something of a two-headed experience when it comes to allowing imperfection. I know that sounds weird, humour me while I explain. I want this book to be good enough for you and good enough for me. Good enough to connect with you, to be good enough to translate my inner world to the outer world, be good enough to tell my experiences of living with the curse of too much and not enough, and to give you good enough chances to be held in pockets of rest while your brain and body mull over your own narrative of too much and not enough. I want it to be flippin' excellent. I want readers to say:

'Damn, Sarah Wheeler wrote a freakin' brilliant book.'

Why do I want that? Because I grew up trying to make sure that my writing was the best. I wanted to impress my teacher and get A grades because that was the name of the game in school. Be the best, and even if one's work was the best, there were always ways to improve. The messaging was clear: never be complacent or satisfied with what had been accomplished. Anything below an A grade was unacceptable. There was no hint that maybe the C-grade essay was, in fact, enough, good enough. Everything about school was about comparison. I was always checking with myself to see if I was better than her/better than him, knowing I would never be as good at writing as her. Six years after leaving school, I sat in a training session held by the tutoring company I worked for, and we watched a speech by a teacher and conductor named Benjamin Zander. If you are a teacher, stop reading this and go watch his 'Everybody Gets an A' speech online. Zander enthusiastically explains to a gaggle of bored-looking, dumbfounded headteachers that every student deserves an A or at least they should start with being given an A because then that young person will believe they are able to achieve an A. The student would make an effort because they believe in themselves instead of trying to survive and outdo their peers. I loved what he was saying. I wished my teachers had been Zandered, but I still maintain, after working with loads of stressed-out teenagers, that it is totally OK to be satisfied with good enough rather than perfect. Done is as valid as perfect. So, while writing in my journal and scrappy bits of paper, including napkins and sticky notes, I caught myself a lot of times going down the perfectionism tunnel. Is there a better adjective I could use? More lyrical ways to describe? Is my vocabulary choice suitably varied? My inner dialogue resembled the comments left in red pen by teachers on essays.

Turns out that book writing is a transformational process, plus a headfuck for the voices of perfectionism. I panicked that I am not intelligent enough to write about the things I want to write about. I am not a medical professional, not a mental health expert, no historian, no scientist, no Feminist critic, no scholarly authority on the origins of patriarchy. What if my ideas and words do not match up with the women who have written before me and will write after me, women who are 'proper authors' with huge followings and publishing houses clamouring to buy their next book? Everything I write must be expertly put together, researched, fabulously eloquent, and measured, else I will sound amateur or, Goddess forbid, like some angry woman mouthing off about everything that has made her body, mind, and heart go from peaceful to rageful to recovered and back again a million times over. It dawned on me that I had labelled myself as an unskilled, too-much nobody with nothing important to say. My head hung, my shoulders hunched and my energy lulled. *Who am I to write this?* It was this familiar somatic reaction which sent me right back to school, trying to get all the answers right with the highest grade so I could be the best, win the praise and breathe a sigh of relief for avoiding being exposed as a talentless fraud once again, until the next homework was due. I am imperfect. Who wants to hear from an imperfect person?

The classist, intelligence-fetishizing world we inhabit reveres experts. Patriarchy reveres male experts and gives bloody hell to women who raise their hearts and voices to be heard. I remembered my witch who was throttled for being herself, cast out for living how she wanted to live. I was frightened when I lived as a witch, frightened as a child in school, and frightened now. I remembered my witch and my tears came screaming out, pouring down my face as I sat in bed on a rainy day, compulsively hitting the keys on my laptop. I am no expert and I am writing anyway. Fuck it.

The imperfect is where we begin, and imperfect is where we may wish to stay. Even though alchemists turn base metals into gold, I believe that the shiny end product is not the whole story. I have a hunch that alchemists were spellbound by the process, the transformation of transmutation, as they returned to their process time and again. Alchemists rarely found their gold, it was elusive, just like perfection. Maybe they were looking in the wrong places for their elixirs? The process is where the gold is if we can only allow our process to be imperfect. I am letting my writing process be imperfect. My heart lit up when I typed that sentence! When it comes to patriarchy's standards, I do not have it all together. I am on the supposedly wrong side of thirty-five, I am not thin, I am not rich but realise I have socioeconomic privilege that I have not earned because I am white, I am not a parent and have no desire to be, I have no steady job as yoga teaching is part of the gig economy, I bleed heavily each month and do not pretend that I don't, my laughter has been labelled 'too loud' and so have my tears. I still live with symptoms of PTSD, which my ex told me 'makes me a mess'. Yep, sometimes I am a mess, and I reserve the right to my messiness because recovery is messy. (Messiness is all good as long as we and nobody else are being harmed by the messiness).

We are not given permission to be imperfect. So I granted myself this permission. So much about this book will be imperfect because that is who I am. Proudly imperfect. Give yourself the permission. We will find the path together as we untangle from the grip of perfection under patriarchy's curse. Let your reading of this book be imperfect, dip in and out, take your rest. I just want you to be able to breathe.

Go slowly now. Inhale, exhale, inhale, exhale, inhale, exhale. Repeat.

Rising

Find a photograph of yourself where you perceive yourself as imperfect. Frame it and put it where you can see it.

Write for a couple of minutes on each prompt …

When was the first time you recall trying to be perfect?

What do you experience in your body when you remember this time?

As a child, what messages did you soak up regarding perfection?

In the next chapter, we will explore how the seeds of too much and not enough are sown in women from an early age, planting patterns of 'must try harder' which grow into subtle subservience, to bending over backwards to help everybody but ourselves.

Rest.

Cross The Threshold,

Peer Into Your Dark To See Your Light.

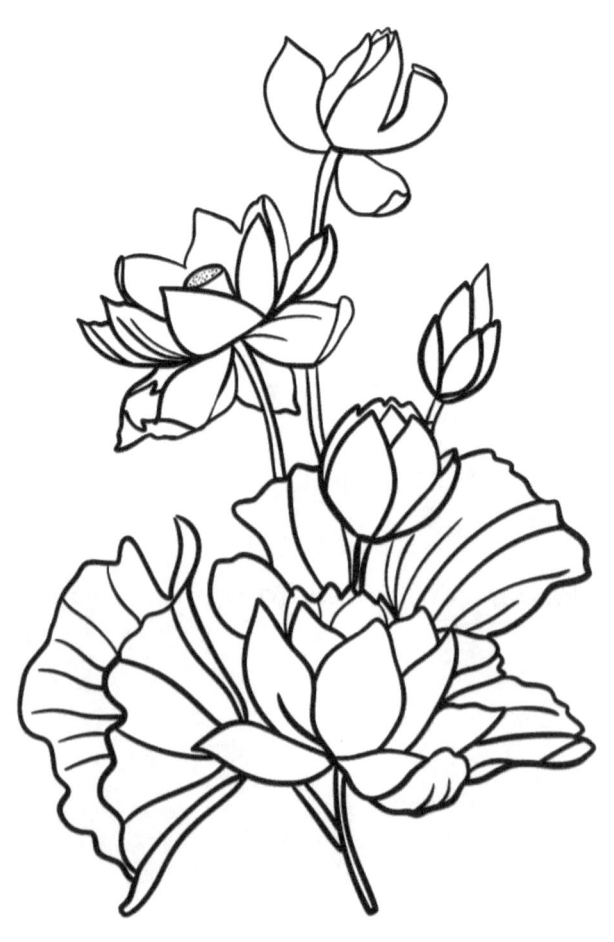

CHAPTER EIGHT

Busy Girls and Good Girls

Rest

Take some time out for yourself with this chapter's guided rest practice in the *Enough!* area at youreenoughyoga.com.

Recovery

Hands up, who found school bloody hard? The education system offers a ton of opportunity to come face to face with the curse of too much and not enough, especially if you happen to be a girl. A fly on the wall back in the late 90s would be forgiven for thinking that I was sailing through high school; A grades in everything apart from maths – which I was failing miserably, a group of friends, thankfully no relentless bullying but only brief run-ins with a couple of the school bullies, a social life of trips into town mainly to window shop the hallowed grounds of Topshop and Miss Selfridge (I felt a pang of nostalgia for my teenage shopping habits when Topshop, my former playground, closed its real-life stores this year thanks to bloody Covid). I was doing well (on paper) in a school system that, in the 90s, certainly did not care for the wellbeing of students. Truth be told, several of my friends and I were nervous wrecks during high school. Why? Because puberty is the worst thing ever and is made even more unbearable thanks to society's refusal to hold open, unabashed conversations about the female-heavy topics like the menstrual cycle, or how to empower girls to recognise abusive behaviour and misogyny, and of course, the enormous elephant in the room named patriarchy, which pathologises and objectifies the female body even more oppressively when girls reach puberty. I used to roll up my school skirt because I wanted to attract male attention. I'm not going to lie about that, but what I was not wise to was that short skirts were not a prerequisite for commanding respect from peers of the opposite sex. With every roll of my skirt, my teen self thought I would be more popular. Little did I know that I was blindly following the structure of a society that wants women to gift-wrap ourselves for the reward of male attention. I did not know that attention is not the same as respect. Hindsight is a wonderful thing, hey? If I could go back in time, I would whisper in my own 13-year-old ear, *Roll up your skirt if you want, babe, that's your choice and your right, but I promise it will earn you zero respect from blokes. Roll down a couple of skirt layers and make friends with yourself. You're enough with a skirt to your ankles and enough with it just covering your bum.*

Being Schooled for Not Enoughness

Puberty is hard for girls (yes, yes, I know it's tough for boys too), but school makes it harder. Do you remember being tired when you came home from school? Or so tired that you struggled to get up on time to dash to the school bus? The UK school day starts too early and finishes too late. Teenagers need way more sleep than adults because their bodies are going through an inordinate amount of change. Sleep is when the body restores itself and replenishes energy reserves, not to mention giving the brain a chance to go offline from wakeful busyness and indulge in relaxation along with dreaming, which helps the brain to file events and make sense of our waking lives. Again, thank fuck I was not a teen with a smartphone ready to distract me into scrolling at any opportunity, rich with apps with algorithms to profit from holding my attention online for longer. Facebook does not care if it is stealing sleep from teenagers; it is designed to keep any user hooked, regardless of whether it is time for lights out and rest. So by the time morning rolls around, teens are tired because they need a longer sleep anyhow, plus they have had to part company with their online life in enough time to get proper rest, and they have to wake up to start a school day with classroom time kicking off before 9 am. The school day crams in at least five lessons per day plus homework, plus after-school team sports and extracurricular activities, should the teen want to attend. It is the same grind every damn day.

The vibe in my school towards productivity, effort, and attainment was clear. You better be doing your absolute best, but even your best may not be good enough because your classmate's best might be better. It was academic competition all day, every day. Tired teenagers being cajoled to do their best which ultimately may not be enough because the world is competitive. A close friend of mine who is a high school teacher told me that the need for students to compete with peers is promoted all day, there is no break from it, while teachers are encouraged to compete with other teachers. School taught me and my peers that we better be ready for a life of proving ourselves because there will always be somebody who can outperform you. If you got an A this time, why not get an A* next time? More to the point, why didn't you get an A* this time? You can do better. Better, better, must do better, nothing was ever enough in school. If you're on the B team for netball, why not aim for the A team? Never enough. Even when I slogged my guts out to get an A in my science GCSE, my teacher did not believe me when I proudly showed him my grades slip:

'Are you sure, Sarah? You're not making a mistake, are you?'

A teacher pulled me aside one day and said he noticed I had been off school a few times in the last couple of months and he snootily questioned me about why I was missing school. I immediately felt ashamed. I used to get headaches and wrecking tummy cramps around my period and frankly needed to rest, so I would take a day off here and there. I never felt guilty for it up until then. But the teacher thought he knew best and said that I would miss crucial teaching for the exams and my grades would suffer if I kept missing school. *Shit, maybe he is right. Better power on through,* I thought. *Maybe I am asking for too much by taking time to rest?* Wish I could go back in time and tell him to mind his damn business.

Busy Woman in Training

School is so full-on, so entrenched in messaging to fulfil one's potential. Latin maxims embroidered on school uniforms: *Carpe Diem.* Rinse and repeat. This is when mainstream school can be harmful to girls, steering us away from listening to what our energy levels need. Nobody in school was ever talking about the fact that female energy can nosedive dramatically in the lead-up to a period and be accompanied by myriad symptoms such as anxiety, low mood, and tension headaches. Girls are simply not designed to do the same thing day after day, the same school routine, homework routine, sports team routine, eating routine. The lack of awareness awarded by the education system to the physical needs of girls and their cycles is the training ground for the world of work which demands that women slay it at work every day, regardless of what our bodies need from us. School trains women to relentlessly produce results offering zero compassion to ourselves to tune into what type of work may be more suited to our cycle at any time of the month. Exerting our effort for the A* grade in a few years morphs into exerting our effort to work the hardest and longest, possibly for a promotion (or maybe not because men are promoted more often than women). Nothing wrong with working hard, but the systems we live in do not cater for the female landscape, which changes from week to week, whether a woman still bleeds or follows the moon cycles after menopause.

I hear from friends who chose the thankless career of teaching within the mainstream (State) school system that things are changing; students are actively encouraged to be aware of mental health issues like anxiety, depression, and the triggers for these illnesses, such as cyberbullying and peer pressure. It is good news that the school system is waking up to the importance of nurturing teen mental health. But something tells me that the school system itself starts to make girls sick from inside the system as schools churn out swathes of young women who have been worked for six hours per day (excluding homework or extracurricular activities) with no regard for whether this is the right time of their cycle to be working so hard. I absolutely think that girls should pursue the highest grades, but only if that is what they truly want. If I had believed that I was enough with or without the A grades or with or without enough exam points as my passport to higher education, I would never have pushed myself so hard. Perhaps I would have been satisfied with a string of

Bs and better mental health. I would love to go back in time and tell teen Sarah:

'Listen, it is a savvy plan to aim high, but as you grow, you will see that life has so much more to offer, and you have so much more to offer than a bunch of letters on your grade slip.'

This way, we might empower young women to believe that they are more than a commodity that can only vouch for her worth with a few letters on a piece of paper. Patriarchy loves commodification. The system wants to see what women have to offer (which is obviously loads) but also what it can take from us – again, loads. Patriarchy wants women who are perfect packages, commodified on LinkedIn profiles as evidence for their intelligence, schooling, a Russell Group or Ivy League university, with skills to be offered up to careers that will pay them less than men and frown upon their choice to procreate (or not) then chew up their energy and spit them out, especially if women work for institutions like the NHS or the police service. One day there will be a LinkedIn profile that reads:

'This is me. Take it or leave it. I am enough either way. PS, Fuck the system.'

Dramas

If we are privileged enough, we get our grades that allow us to trot off to university. I never wanted to be on an academic university course because I had always wanted to go to drama school. I didn't need high grades because entry to acting courses was based on passing auditions, an early insight into ruthless, rejection-heavy showbiz. Looking back, it is both no accident and utterly astounding that I, somebody who was convinced I would never be good enough, wanted to forge myself into the most competitive rejection-heavy career on the planet. The acting business is a constant barrage of shit from the curse of too much and not enough, and unsurprisingly, women bear the brunt of this barrage. I stood in castings, hearing directors openly talk about fellow female auditionees as if they were not there: 'Number two is too tall, number five just does not look right,' et cetera. A woman I went with to an audition training class left the room in tears because the male tutor told her she would need to lose about 10 pounds if she wanted to get on TV. She was around a UK size 10. Her dress size is not the point. How fucking dare he tell her what to do with her body? That night she and I went out dancing, drank so much vodka until we threw up in a gutter, cussing the guy into the middle of next week. Secretly I worried that it would not be long until somebody told me to lose weight so I'd better up my exercise; the showbiz industry and anorexia are not a healthy combination.

I understand now that I wanted to go to drama school because I wanted to play at being other people. I had loved drama classes at school. Reading scripts was time to take on a character, connecting with emotions that I felt were too much, unacceptable for me to feel in my real life, but were somehow safer in the guise of a character. Perhaps that's why we watch soap operas: to see the emotional spectrum displayed for us from inside a screen without us having to feel into our own pain. There was also the persona of an actor, which was attractive to me. I decided it needed to comprise confidence, outgoingness, being personable, walking into audition rooms and looking like I had everything together. After leaving drama school, I would attend auditions in my actor persona. I would show that I wanted the part but I did not need the part. Except, of course, I did always need those parts because A) I really needed the money, and B) because a new role would mean another escape into being somebody else.

The showbiz industry is harsh, particularly for young women. During auditions for drama school and when looking for agency representation, there was an industry truth (not even an unspoken truth!) that there will always be another young female actor who will be better than you, more talented, so you better be your best every damn day while becoming a pro at getting rejected. I remember the tutor's speech from one of my drama school auditions:

'This course will take everything from you and so will the business. You will be tired every day and then you will need to go to work after class to pay your bills. I expect to see you working as well as attending this course.'

At least he was honest.

'I want to see people who can show me the truth in every performance.'

High expectations, plus when it comes to critiquing a performance, it is all so subjective, so who says what truth is anyway? Wish I had cottoned on to that when I was doing the audition rounds. Drama school had nothing to offer when it came to dealing with the inevitable hurt of continual rejection, nor how to care adequately for one's mental health so that actors can bounce back and look for the next bit of work. A writing sister of mine, Natalie Farrell, is an author, presenter, and singer and recalls her entry into showbiz and the exhaustion of her training:

'I came out of music college absolutely depleted. I just lost every sense of confidence. I did not want to sing. I did not want to do anything. I was on the floor. Where was the pastoral care? This was the time when I most experienced being too much and not enough.'

These days, Natalie has flipped the script of exhaustion and not-enoughness within her soul-led work of empowering people to truly dance with life to find sanctuary in their own hearts. She also creates beautiful soul-infused music.

We need more people like Natalie! Imagine having a teacher like her in school.

While I was a student at drama school, I was only capable of less-than-entry-level self-care, partly due to being eighteen years old, partly due to having never heard of self-care, and partly due to the fierce competition between the other young women in my year who all wanted the validation of teachers and peers alike. We had to be at our best, putting on a show every day so that we might be noticed for the next round of castings. Except it was never enough because we were always being told we could do better. One of the acting tutors literally said about my class:

'You're all good but you can all be better.' Good was not enough.

Anybody who attends a performing arts college after high school will certainly be having a unique experience of the higher education system. Compared to friends who were studying more academic courses, my degree in acting was gruelling with its 9 am-7 pm timetable, while those on history or English degrees had a few hours of lectures each week. Even though academic courses have fewer hours of bums on seats in lectures, it does not mean that academically minded students do not feel the pressure to get the highest grades. Students skip sleep to study in the library late into the night, party super hard because of FOMO and buy non-prescribed drugs to enhance their concentration and productivity (Adderall is a college fave in the USA). The reality is that getting a high college score will never fill the hole called *I am not enough*. Fabulous achievements and accolades may plug the hole for a while, but without a baseline of knowing you are enough with or without a degree, the hole still exists. If we experienced feeling that we were not enough as small children when we struggled with our three times table (like I did), or because our sibling was afforded more attention by a parent, our grown-up selves will not be able to remedy that not-enoughness with a First-Class Honours Degree. Plus, for women, patriarchy has conned us into believing we are both too much and not enough, so we are damned if we aim high and damned if we don't.

The education system under patriarchy demands that women perform at all costs, that we fight with each other and with the sheer volume of studying and tests required from us when we are simply not designed for peak performance all day, every day. Our cycles mean we are not designed for constant productivity, but the system demands it. The mainstream education system does not make space to foster the cyclical lifestyle that women really need; instead, it normalises depletion. What young women need to be educated in (among many things that the current model does not provide!) is the development and nurturing of a foundational belief that she is enough no matter what, she is enough if her schoolwork improves and enough if it does not. That she is not too much for having emotions that have been deemed unpalatable such as anger, grief, sadness, or jealousy. Our girls also need to be shown how to rest. With rest as a touchstone in a woman's life, she can choose to opt out of what she does not really want to be doing in favour of rest, or on the flipside, slay it at every available opportunity because she has taken enough rest to kick ass without depletion.

I Promise to Be a Good Girl

School is not the only place where girls get trained to follow patriarchal conditioning. When I was seven, I started going to Brownies. I loved it because on Brownie night, my best friend would come over for tea and then we would walk up to the church hall together for the evening's jolly frolics. Many a Brownie meeting was spent doing wholesome, useful stuff like learning to make a cup of tea, learning semaphore (slightly more interesting than making tea) and sewing, before the evening would descend into enjoyable organised chaos as 35 girls all under twelve ran around the church hall playing a game not dissimilar to British Bulldogs.

My bestie and I would laugh uncontrollably while playing games and singing weird songs. I was not a boisterous child and didn't feel the impulse to ever deliberately behave badly for the fun of winding up adults. In fact, I was a shy child but I still felt the repetitive sting of being made so aware day in and day out at school that stepping out of line, not waiting my turn, or questioning the point of certain activities were traits that were frowned upon. As a child, I do not remember ever feeling autonomous or brave enough to say, no, I did not want to do something. I was reserved and didn't play up at home or school, so Brownies felt like a safe space to be around other girls of my age, be silly and raucous, and I know this really coaxed me out of my shell. However, looking back, I cannot help but think critically about the narrative of well-loved institutions like the Guiding Association. There was some questionable groupthink, behaviour control, and patriarchal propaganda touted at Brownies in the 1990s, and some of this groupthink still underpins the movement, perpetuating the curse of too much and not enough.

Hang on while I put my non-expert historian hat on. Lord Robert Baden- Powell was the founder of the Scouts, which later added a group for girls called the Guides. Baden Powell and his wife, Olave, believed in outdoorsy education for young people and provided youth groups where teens could enjoy camping, building dens and orienteering (for the Boy Scouts) and cooking, sewing, and other household tasks plus a bit of camping (for the Girl Guides). The original marketing materials for the Girl Guides, founded by Baden Powell's sister Agnes, needed to convince families that their girls would not be 'led astray'. Heaven forbid they end up like those pesky suffragettes. The Guiding Association declared that girls needed to learn how to cope by tooling up with various skills should they end up living in the 'farthest-flung parts of the British empire' in the absence of servants, doctors or trained help.[1] Vomit.

The original Guiding Association was a blend of light female empowerment with a flavour of white colonialism. The Baden Powells were big fans of the concept of Empire. While recalling my time in the Brownies, piecing together the group's maxims with the moulding of helpful little girls, I had a creeping hunch that something rotten may have been at the heart of the founder's designs for the Scouting Movement – all of the patriotism, being healthy and fit, camping trips and outdoor skills, being useful and prepared. I shit you not that a phrase popped into my mind while I awoke at 8 am, mulling over this part of the book: *Hitler Youth*. A Google search for *Baden Powell Racist* sadly confirmed my morning hunch in less than one second. Lord BP was an ardent admirer of Hitler and his fascist leanings. Yep, old BP enjoyed a flick through *Mein Kampf*, summarising it in a 1939 diary entry as 'a wonderful book, with good ideas on education, health, propaganda, organisation'. In 1937 BP met the Nazi-German Ambassador in London to compare notes on how their youth organisations were run, with a view for the 'Scouts to come into closer touch with the youth movement in Germany'. Apparently, the Nazis were anxious to forge a Hitler Youth/Scouting collaboration. Baden-Powell and Hitler never met in person (thank fuck) but continued to share rotten ideals. When one of BP's German Scout leaders was forced to a concentration camp, BD was non-plussed because the leader was homosexual, and so according to fascism-approving BP, this discrimination was the correct move.[2] So there we have it – the founder of the Scouting Movement, from which sprung the Guides and Brownies, was an unapologetic, Nazi-friendly, racist homophobe.

At Brownies, I believe I was being trained to become a good girl. Being good meant being cheerful and obedient while habitually doing stuff for other people and ignoring one's own needs. Girls who were not cheerful and obedient were too much and not enough. There were badges to earn to prove you were enough. These badges proved your productivity levels to show how much good stuff you had done, or what skill deemed useful by the Brownie Handbook you had demonstrated to a high enough standard by the Tester (still sounds creepy almost 30 years later!) to be deemed worth a badge. The Handbook of the 1990s read like a behaviour guide for how to be accepted as a girl in society. The bottom line was roughly, *be good, don't be a nuisance, do your best no matter what and keep your uniform clean.*

Do not get me wrong, I learned some cool things at Brownies and look back on Brownie camping trips to dingy, rainy campsites with fondness. There is something very special about having a space purely for young girls to bond over activities that these days do not have so much emphasis on the home (yes, there were Hostess and Home Skills badges) but include areas such as Mindfulness, Rights, and Zero Waste. However, the historic religious foundations of the Brownies reveal patriarchal structural control and expectations upon women, which still in the 21st century perpetuate the depletion rather than the nurturing of women's energy. These expectations made so clear for children in the Brownies can create models of behaviour and thought suppression, which are detrimental throughout puberty, with damage still being played out when ex-Brownies like me arrived in our mid-thirties! Writing this passage, I literally just stopped to wonder whether my time being told how to act and think in the Brownies contributed to my attraction to joining a group in my early twenties which I later discovered to be a cult …

In Brownies, I made a promise to serve God, my Queen and country, and to always think of others before myself. I remember the ceremony as if it were yesterday, a sure sign that this was a pivotal moment in my formative years. It was a swearing-in ceremony for good girls. All the other girls stood in a massive circle to witness the ceremony. One of the older Brownies held my hand and we skipped around the circle and then into the centre to the sound of the other girls singing a lilting ditty. I had to stand by a sculpture of a large red and white spotted toadstool which I now recognise as the Amanita Muscaria fungus (a type of magic mushroom). I had to recite my vow to serve God, my Queen and country in front of the leader of the Brownie pack, known as Brown Owl. Reading this back to myself while I write, this all sounds super weird and straight out of *The Wicker Man!*

If there were a Good Girl Manifesto, the Brownie Promises and Laws (yes, they seriously call their guiding principles a Law) would be it. At age seven, I promised to always put other people before myself and to always 'lend a hand'. On reflection, this promise bred hordes of little rescuers, eager beavers too keen to help others, perhaps to the detriment of the rescuers' own needs and boundaries. To this day, when I attend therapy, I hold space for my ingrained belief that I am not enough, not important to people if I am not useful, while recovering from compulsive helpfulness. Things have changed in the Guiding Association now, and young people no longer have to promise to serve God, nor do UK Scouts. Sadly, the Boy Scouts of America do not allow atheist or agnostic members. This is a relief because the God which is referred to is the male interpretation of God, and it is sinister to think of little girls promising to serve him. I thought it was totally weird for me to say I wanted to serve that God when I was making my Brownie Promise over 30 years ago, but I didn't question it. I believed it was what I had to do. Girl Guides now pledge to be true to themselves, develop their beliefs and serve their monarch and country (Girl Guide Promise, 2014). This is an improvement, but let's take a breath because promising to serve the monarch remains problematic. The monarch is the head of the Church of England and is responsible for appointing clergy in the upper hierarchy of the Church. The Church of England believe pretty damn strongly that God is male, so was it even worth the Guiding Association removing the religious aspect of the promises taken by young girls if they still must serve the monarch, who represents the highest order of the Church? Maybe I am making a tenuous link here, what do you think?

I can't help but remember high school history, where we learned that British monarchs are automatically made head of the Church. This mash-up of religion and royalty began with misogynist extraordinaire Henry VIII, who declared himself God's top dog, appointing himself as the first monarch to be head of the Church, in a stroke of self-serving shadiness because he needed those divorces! Perhaps by serving the monarch, Girl Guides serve God by proxy? Perhaps the subtext is that a girl who does not serve the monarch is not doing enough for her country, that being a good woman means being patriotic. Perhaps one becomes unruly, chaotic (too much!) without a framework to serve her monarch? I'm thinking out loud here, you may completely disagree and say I am reading too much into these connected dots of patriarchal church, monarchy, and organised youth groups. My gut tells me I am on to something. Whatever your feelings on the interconnectedness of God and monarchy and young people pledging allegiance to one or both, the paradox remains: 'It's not appropriate to ask children to pledge allegiance to a head of state. You can't be true to yourself and your conscience and pledge allegiance to one person; it contradicts itself.' A point well made by Graham Smith of the anti-monarchy group 'Republic', cited in *The Independent*, 2013.

I do not regret going to Brownies and I know my parents had the best intentions for sending me, and I always remember leaving Brownie night laughing and smiling. But I would have given it a miss had I known about the founder's appreciation of a totalitarian despot. Sure I did not know about fascism when I was seven, but I knew Hitler was bad news. However, Brownie fun and games aside, due to my formative years of indoctrination to serve others before myself, I developed patterns that needed to be healed, patterns which underpinned my quality of life for many years and left me exhausted, always trying to do my best, serve others and think of others before myself (luckily I gave up caring about the monarchy ages ago!). I realise things are different at Brownies now, but the Brownies I experienced in the 1990s trained girls to be subservient, useful little helpers. As a grown-up, within my work, relationships, and self-image, it was as if I still needed to earn badges to sew onto an invisible Brownie sash, proving myself to be at my best day after day, those little triangular badges boosting my self-esteem.

Rising

What would you change, improve or scrap altogether from our current education system?

Do you agree or disagree with how children are educated in the mainstream system? Why?

What do our little girls need to know?

What would you tell your little self about working hard and competition?

What kind of anti-Brownie ceremony would you like to hold for your younger self? What promises would you make to yourself?

Do you remember the first time you felt exhausted after school or extra-curricular activities? What happened? What did you need?

What good girl training did you receive and from who?

Do you believe that any effort you make is enough?

What you witnessed and learned while growing up will have so much to say about your opinion of yourself as an adult. It is so crucial that we teach our girls that:

They are not productivity machines.

Other women are not competition.

They are enough whether they are getting As or Fs at school.

They do not need to help out at every opportunity.

AND they have ultimate jurisdiction over the sacred ground that is their body.

It was etched onto her Body,

Every detail.

Things to remind her,

A scent of beer and cigs,

Sweat,

An airless apartment,

Generic cologne on a striped sweater,

Etched onto her Body.

It was etched onto her body,

Every detail.

Things to remind her,

Her tears, her fight,

Her courage, her falling, her rising.

Etched onto her Body.

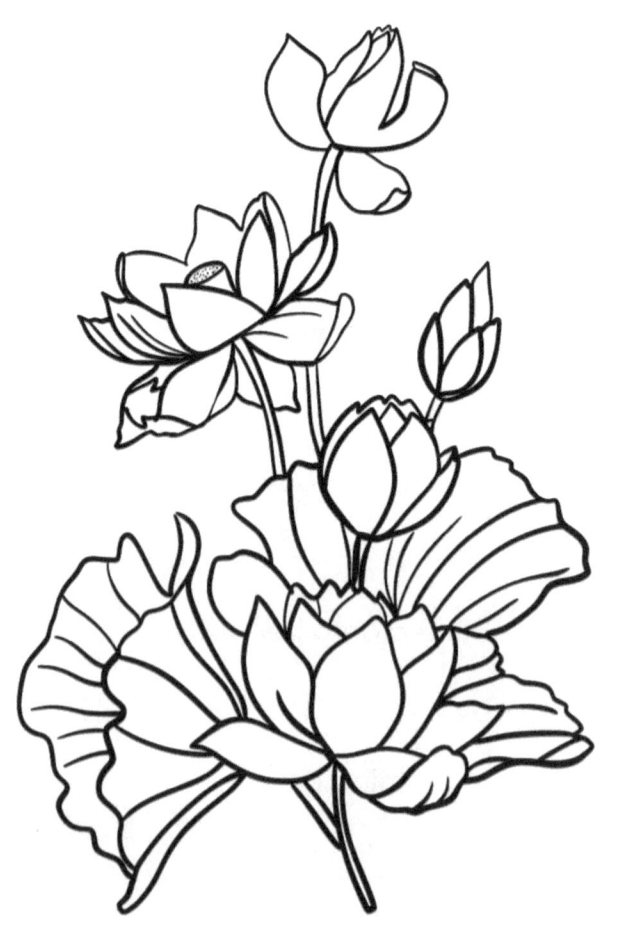

CHAPTER NINE

Body

Rest

Shimmy over to the *Enough!* area at youreenoughyoga.com for this chapter's Yoga Nidrā practice. This one is infused with the energy of the rose.

Recovery

Patriarchy teaches women that our bodies are both too much and not enough. This myth manifested within my troubling relationship with my own body. My body has been a place where I have abused myself and a place that others have abused. It has been touched with love but also violation. My body has ingested substances that were damaging, but this body of mine has also been nourished by delicious, wholesome foods, it has been the site of much pleasure and untold pain. My body and I have had an on/off relationship because I believed patriarchy's propaganda. They feed us an impossible body-based to-do list: *be willowy but not too tall, be thin but have curves in the right places, get toned but not muscular, be blonde but make it look natural, keep your skirt short but don't wear it outdoors, show us your cleavage but don't disappoint us when the Wonderbra comes off, lose the body hair apart from the porn strip for your pubes, have a few drinks with us but don't act drunk, order dessert so long as you hit the gym the next day, carry our babies but lose the weight fast but be ready to get knocked up again whenever we want, wear your high heels but do not tower over me.*

Hot is Subjective

Patriarchy thinks it owns the female body. They like to tell us their opinions about our form and what to do to rectify faults that they pick. In sixth form, I remember hearing two boys comparing the girls' tits: Girl A doesn't have enough up top, while Girl B has nice tits but has rolls on her stomach. The boys wished these girls could swap body parts while the boys mentally built their own Barbies. For a long time, I bought into these proprietorial notions that the female body simply exists to attract a man because I thought the path to happiness came in the shape of a partner, a man in my case. On unconscious but sometimes very conscious levels, I did what I thought I needed to do with this body of mine to win the man who I thought would save me from myself. I believed that if I found him and, most importantly, could keep him around, all the hate I had inflicted on myself would puff into thin air. I starved myself, harmed myself, drugged myself, and consensually let myself be fucked by unpleasant men because I thought these were the rules of engagement. Truthfully, although I was saying yes to all of this, it was not really what I wanted. *Do what the man wants you to do and you will win him*, says society. It doesn't work. What happened to me instead was self-abandonment, addiction and a piss-poor set of boundaries. He won't stay if you mould yourself into what he wants. He will get bored when he has conquered your body and run out of steam to love-bomb you with, no matter how hot you dress or how hot you fuck or how hot you keep your body. Plus, 'hot' is subjective and all too often dictated by men who grew up on jazz mags in the 70s, porn in the 80s, *FHM* in the 90s, and the modern medium of Instagram and Snapchat where girls get pressured into sending nudes to boy classmates to gain approval.

Patriarchy has rules about more than what we should do with or what we let other people do to our bodies. Patriarchy thinks it rules the appearance of the female form. Let me widen the net once more, though, and note that society seems to think that everybody's body should be thin, regardless of gender. Women, men, non-binary and trans people all have the right to give our collective middle finger to society regarding the norms that dictate what sizes and shapes are acceptable. No matter who you are, it is nobody's fucking business what weight you are now or what weight you choose to be. Thing is, I am a woman and I have lived and breathed the impact of what this male-favouring society thinks it can decree about my body. It is etched on my body. Society is fat-phobic toward all genders, but it is women who bear the brunt of this body/weight dictatorship. Patriarchy grants no space for the nuances that a woman's body cycles through and gives no wriggle room for the changes which happen to the female body as we age. Patriarchy teaches us to be obsessed with decreasing our weight and denying our ageing. If a man has a beer belly and grey hair society is much less judgemental of him than of the woman who dares to show a rotund stomach at the beach or flaunt her flowing silver hair. The rules of the sixth-form boys still apply; it is the woman who must preen to attract the man while the man is afforded a viewing platform to judge the woman's efforts. *Good luck,* says society, if you are an older, fat, greying woman. *The scrapheap is waiting for you.* Unsurprisingly though, Western culture has it all twisted.

A couple of thousand years ago, it was accepted for women to be large all over, all soft round curves, wide behind and voluptuous boobs. Figurines of women found in archaeological sites, such as the figure nicknamed 'The Venus of Willendorf', show the shape of the Goddess. She was round, proud and desired. I like to imagine that Venus did not give one solitary shit about what people thought of her body. I wish I thought like her. Fat shaming is rife, and something tells me Venus would not have stood for it. The assumption reinforced by the media is that all women want to be thin and young, and if women are not hunting down these so-called desirable ideals, then, again, good luck and enjoy the scrapheap. The Goddess disagrees. She longs for us to be compassionate toward the body we each have because seated in the body is the connection to the Earth, the sacred ground which seeded us and keeps us rooted. She wants us to embrace the size and shape we are but feel free to make changes for OURSELVES, not as a result of a patriarchy's anti-fat messaging. If women do not authentically want to lose pounds purely for themselves then everybody else can just back the fuck off, leaving women to be our desired size. The same goes if women are authentically happy being thin. Let fat women be fat and let thin women be thin. Let aging women age. End of.

Patriarchy's Medical Establishment

Unfortunately, in the West, we have a medical system which grossly underfunds research into woman-centred medicine while also basing assessments of a 'healthy body' on the male body. Therefore, patriarchy seeps into the medical establishment's assessment of what is deemed healthy for women's bodies. It is known that the medical establishment reduces women's pain to psychosomatic or pure hypochondria, particularly when women present with symptoms of cell damage as in ME/CFS (myalgic encephalomyelitis/chronic fatigue syndrome). Rather than examining why women are four times as likely as men to have ME/CFS or Lyme disease, these illnesses are shoved into the shadows and ridiculed as being all in the head. Julie Nausbam from the Long Island School of Medicine was quoted in *The Guardian*:

'In general, there's not as much research money and attention on conditions that primarily affect women. That's just a general disparity in medical research. I think certain biases persist that when women present with a lot of body aches or pains, there's more often an emotional or personality component to it than medical origin.'

The medical establishment, ruled over by CDC and big pharma, attempted to ruin the career of scientist Judy Mikovits when she purported that there may be a link between the pre-existing human retroviruses in the body which may cause the onset of ME/CFS due to immune dysfunction possibly triggered by vaccinations. Caveat from me: you do not have to subscribe to either germ theory (the currently accepted scientific theory that germs invade the body and cause a number of diseases) or terrain theory (the idea that viruses do not exist, that it is our environment, from the emotional to the physical, and our level of toxicity which causes disease) to accept that the patriarchal medical establishment really tried to screw Judy over.

She was incarcerated (yes, she did actual jail time) thanks to the collaboration of big players in big pharma, including Tony Fauci, for speaking publicly about her theory and the results she was finding from her research into retroviruses and vaccines. For trying to validate and understand the causation of the legitimate diagnosis of ME/CFS for all sufferers, she was shut down and ostracised by the scientific community. This was because she dared to research the scientific taboos of ME/CFS and vaccines, even more courageously speaking out about a possible link between these two taboos. If you want to read a true story of pure patriarchy, check out Mikovits' book called Plague, which explores the whole sorry affair.

I'm going to go off topic but still kinda on topic for a minute and mention the global headfuck that is Covid and its impact on women's bodies. Women are getting screwed over by the disease, along with the global response to controlling and treating it. Women are more likely than men to develop long Covid, as is the case with other post-viral syndromes.[1] Perhaps this is because women have faced epidemic levels of underlying health issues exacerbated by trauma and chronic stress, putting their long-term recovery from Covid at risk due to the strain already shouldered by the female body. *The Lancet* medical journal reported that women are disproportionately affected by the social and economic impact of Covid.[2] This is due to government-imposed, unpopular lockdown policies. Lockdowns stop people working and take kids out of schools, the majority of childcare being done by women who need to take time off from work to look after the children, plus throw in the inequality which girls face globally with regard to accessing education. Women are picking up the pieces of the at best, incompetently, at worst, nefariously handled Covid situation. The cherry on this unpleasant cake is that now we can see that women are more impacted by adverse events from the mass Covid jabs. In late 2021, Pfizer released vaccine data documents to lawyer Aaron Siri, who acts on behalf of the Public Health and Medical Professionals for Transparency organisation. Pfizer list and agree in this data that in the first two and a half months of the Emergency Use Authorisation of their Covid jab, 29,914 women suffered adverse events (gastrointestinal, skin disorders, respiratory system disorder, nervous system disorder and thoracic disorders) compared with 9,182 vaccine related adverse events in men.

In even worse news, it has now come to light, thanks to a presentation hosted by The World Council for Health that the Pfizer Covid jab has had a negative impact on women's menstrual cycles.[3] One study revealed that women with endometriosis who took the Pfizer jab saw a worsening in their condition.[4] Where pregnant women are concerned, there is no long-term safety data for the effects of the Covid jabs on this demographic. One study by CANVAS (Canadian National Vaccine Safety Network) shows that:

'Pregnant vaccinated females had an increased odds of a significant health event within 7 days of the vaccine after two doses of Mrna-1273 compared with pregnant unvaccinated controls within the past 7 days.' If I were pregnant, this seems like a roll of the dice I would be unwilling to take.

Given the fact that women are gaslighted on the regular by the medical establishment as to the causes and existence of their illnesses, I would bet that these adverse events recorded in this data set are just the tip of the iceberg. I bet there are many women who are yet to convince a doctor to record and report their jab-related adverse events.

Back to women and weight. Male-centric guidelines formed from male-centric research keep some women trapped on a carousel of diets and over-exercise or unnecessary surgery for way too long. Enter the BS that is the BMI (body mass index). According to the UK's National Health Service website, 'Body mass index is a measure that uses your height and weight to work out if your weight is healthy. The BMI calculation divides an adult's weight in kilograms by their height in metres squared.' I knew of BMI from my time being measured and weighed during referral for treatment for anorexia nervosa. Back then, my BMI was too high (in other words, I was not underweight enough) to warrant the NHS spending money on inpatient care for me, but my BMI was in the lowest region, which informed doctors that there was indeed something physically wrong with me. Never mind what was physically wrong (low blood pressure, fainting, headaches and cramps), the mental struggle I faced on the daily was deemed not enough by the medical establishment for me to receive intensive in-patient care to help me to recover from the eating disorder, because for the medical establishment, physical symptoms trump mental illness every time. In truth, had I been admitted as an in-patient for recovery then I am pretty sure I would have railed against this treatment route as I am not good with strict routine and hate being told what to do. I think the lack of control over what food I would have been encouraged to consume in the hospital would have been far too distressing to me. On the flipside, I know I would have benefitted from more frequent and intense psychotherapy for the underlying wounds which manifested the eating disorder, therapy which is afforded to in-patients. The BMI chart showed that I was not thin enough and, in doctors' opinions, not ill enough to be offered the mental health support which I needed in the early stages of my recovery. There are millions of people suffering with eating disorders who are not offered specialist NHS help for this mental illness because the BMI charts will deem them still inside the 'normal' body mass bracket or in the 'high' body mass bracket. Having a 'normal' or 'high' BMI when being assessed for eating disorder treatment fails to recognise that eating disorders are mental illnesses which are not always symptomised with losing weight or being underweight. If doctors rely too heavily on BMI, then patients are at risk of not receiving the correct diagnosis of an eating disorder and may not be offered adequate care to stimulate their recovery.

The BMI calculation can be misleading where eating disorders are concerned, but the measure can be equally if not more inadequate for assessing whether a woman is indeed overweight. Despite my health being assessed by the supposedly good ol' reliable BMI chart while I was unwell a few years ago, I am a late arrival to the BMI Bullshit Party. While creating this book, I happened across a report on the *Conspirituality* podcast which explored the fact that white supremacy is alive and kicking in health and wellness culture. With a bit more digging, I learned that the formula used for BMI calculation was derived only from the measurement of white male bodies. Yep, BMI does not consider the differences between female to male bodies or perhaps even more sickeningly, BMI is only based on the white body so bears no relationship to what denotes a healthy weight for a person of colour. BMI marginalises women, particularly women of colour, highlighting systemic misogyny and racism within the medical establishment. Alarm bells rang through my body: *Wait, what?! This index is used by mainstream medicine but does not cater to the sizes and shapes of women and non-white folk? Maybe a whole fuck-ton of women from all races have been declared overweight by a system that seems to have been designed for measuring the body mass of mainly European white men??? There must be women walking around thinking they are overweight, falsely labelled by society as lazy and unattractive, women whose bodies have been held out to be inadequate at losing weight that they may not even medically need to lose. Not good enough, too much, taking up too much space.* Women suffering because of spurious information not designed to see us as whole, good, visible, acceptable, enough. I remembered the witches, defamed by false information in religious pamphlets. My heart and mind blown. Fuck patriarchy.

BMI was employed to perpetuate a 19th-century norm called *l'homme moyen* (the average man). In the UK and USA, we have the National Health Service and Centre for Disease Control to thank for continuing to employ this patriarchal, racist weight measurement system in the 21st century. Mainstream medicine has borrowed BMI from the findings of a medically untrained mathematician and astronomer named Lambert Adolphe Jacques Quetelet, who was tasked in the 19th century to find the average levels of obesity among the general population. You might have already guessed that 'general population' meant white men. That's right, women were left out of the research. What a surprise. Quetelet did not design his index to measure an individual's level of fat but focused on what was 'normal' across the population he studied. BMI does not account for the difference in weight between fat and muscle and also ignores the size of an individual's frame. Predictably under the guise of BMI, extremely fit, healthy athletes are dubbed overweight and unhealthy due to the fact that muscle is heavier than fat. If BMI is getting it wrong for athletes, it will be inaccurate for the gym-shy among us too.

The NHS language around their online BMI calculator is problematic. After typing in your weight and height, should you receive the 'healthy weight' result, the site congratulates users by reminding them to 'keep up the good work'. The language chosen subtly implies that those who are not a healthy weight are not doing 'good work' and more subtly, according to the NHS, if one is not in the 'healthy weight' band, one is not 'good'. This implication of healthy = 'good' and unhealthy = 'not good' tied an uneasy, queasy knot in my gut. My gut tells me that the NHS perpetuates non-inclusive ideals represented by Quetelet's work to profile society's average man. If one falls below average, the person is not enough.

Weighing in above average equals a person who is too much. For me, the 'good work' language makes me want to puke as it is yet another reminder that so much of a woman's life is work and measured by work, results that need to be pumped out, all the way down to our precious bodies. As if we don't have enough to do without bringing hard work into the sanctum of how to relate to our bodies. My research into this *l'homme moyen* (the average man) confirmed my queasy gut feeling when I read that Quetelet's *l'homme moyen* profile was used in the 20th century as part of the eugenics movement.[5] Not familiar with eugenics? The Nazis were big fans of this belief system that only wants the fittest and, apparently, best humans to be allowed to procreate. Eugenics aspires to systematically eliminate through sterilisation those who are disabled, poor, neurodivergent and people of colour. Gross.

I don't know if you'd agree, but I think it's time for health services to abandon BMI as a measure of health. BMI is just one way that patriarchy clings to proprietorial oppression of the female body, and the colonisation of the bodies of people of colour. We all know that this is just the tip of a bloody huge iceberg.

Old

How does your body feel when you see or heard the word 'old'? While writing this book, I turned 36. I haven't been particularly concerned about ageing. That was until I saw not one but a flurry of grey hairs protruding from the roots of my hair, winding their way out to make themselves known. I think women who keep their hair long and grey look stunning. Stereotypical as it may sound, there is something wonderfully witchy, powerful, and defiant about women who show off their greys by shunning the dye bottle. So many chemical potions are peddled to us on TV, all promising to give spectacular results to hide the signs of ageing, from greys to laughter lines. I am resolute about living my life on my terms which means knowing I am enough and shaking off the chains of too much. Even with my history of BDD and eating disorder, I have felt determined to resist the pressure to halt the ageing process which is piled upon women. No hiding the greys or laughter lines for me. Or so I thought until I found the little grey rivulets in my roots.

I stood in front of my bathroom mirror. 'Fuck,' I said aloud. Then the tears came. I sobbed quietly, embarrassed by myself for caring about something I had down as so superficial. 'This means I am old.' Something lurched in my stomach, I felt destabilised. 'I am changing,' I thought. I felt scared.

For ten minutes, I examined myself closely in the mirror. Six greys. I'm sure those faint lines were not framing my eyes last week. Lines on the tops of my hands, dry skin around my knuckles. Dimpled skin on my thighs. Are my boobs sagging? Not yet. Phew. Then the stab of insecurity in the centre of my back. What was underneath all this fear? I honestly feel embarrassed to cop to this, but I felt fearful that my partner would leave me because I had begun to age. There, I said it. My partner is younger than me, in his early thirties but looks more like an athlete in his twenties. Everything came at once – fear of being left for a younger specimen, ashamed that ageing might make my bloke stop fancying me, annoyance that I was even having thoughts like these because I try to be kind to myself about my appearance. I resolved to leave the bathroom, get a tea, and hit my journal hard.

It's OK, I am OK, things are OK. I am enough. I am not a loser for worrying about this. This is part of the life cycle. It is normal. Nick loves me and is not a superficial dickhead who will trade me in for a skinny, blonde supermodel.

Soon my panic dropped away and guidance dropped in. *It's patriarchy, you know. All this shame, all this worry about ageing and appearance is the objectification of women and the lack of reverence for our cycles. It is safe to move from Maiden to Mother. It will be safe to move from Mother to Wise Woman to Crone. It's not about me and Nick. It is about the collective fear of the power of the ageing woman and collective fear about Feminine wisdom, her light and her dark.*

Patriarchy is not a fan of the female ageing process. The patriarchal system of control and oppression wants women to stay young. Forget both ageing AND staying youthful. Nope, for patriarchy, it has to be either or. If patriarchy was a man looking for the perfect female mate, he would want his woman to be under forty, under thirty preferably, lithe, tiny waist, large boobs, and no signs of ageing like wrinkles or stretch marks.

If we zoom out from patriarchy and consider Western society in general, we are met with a system which disregards the womanly cycles of life. Unless you grew up with seriously enlightened or pagan caregivers, you may not have heard of the four main cycles of womanhood, these being *Maiden, Mother, Wise Woman* and *Crone*. Ageing is an essential and worthwhile aspect of being alive for all people, and for women, ageing is traditionally represented in the Feminine archetypes of the Wise Woman and the Crone. How does the term Crone make you feel? What images are conjured by this word and its connotations? Honestly, before I began exploring the necessity of embracing each ageing cycle for the sake of my health, all of womankind's health and the whole planet's health, the term Crone conjured up images of a decrepit, wizened, old woman riddled with ailments, to put it bluntly, ugly and past it. We barely see images of old women presented favourably by the media, and unless you had a grandmother who was fully in her power, youthful yet at home with her age and enjoying life as an older person, it is easy to see why the possibility of ageing is not an attractive one. Plus, there is the living trope of the husband who ponces off for an affair with a younger woman. Unfortunately, this well-known scenario reinforces patriarchy's myth that an ageing woman is no longer enough for her male partner, or on the flipside, she becomes too much because blokes have such a poor understanding of the hormonal upheaval of menopause and so they opt for a younger model, one not afflicted by hot flushes and fatigue. This myth about ageing women needs debunking because I learned recently that blokes seeking affairs with younger partners speaks less biologically of the older woman being 'less than' or undesirable, but more accurately speaks to the hormonal changes of the male menopause. Yes, there is such a thing and its proper name is 'andropause'. It was explained to me that men seeking a younger female partner (or male if the ageing man is gay) is connected with the male trying to revisit his youth due to the onset of his own ageing and fatigue (not their partner's), so, in essence, men try to rekindle their own loss of sex drive due to decreased testosterone. Maybe this is why the dudes in the Knights Templar were desperate to find the Holy Grail, the cup to drink from the Fountain of Youth which would restore one to vitality and eternal youth.

Maiden

Let's cycle back, though, if you'll pardon the pun, and explore the earlier cycles: Maiden and Mother. The Maiden is all about youth, virginity. Think willowy teenage girls frolicking joyously around daisy fields on halcyon summer days, scantily dressed, without a care in the world. You can thank the Marc Jacobs advert for Daisy perfume for this homage to the Maiden. We can map this cycle onto the menstrual cycle, so Maiden is the time when energy levels gradually build after the completion of the bleed, perhaps allowing us to feel more sociable, outgoing.

Patriarchy is obsessed with youth and the sexualisation of virginity. It's why we see so many young people on advertising across all kinds of media, as if youth is what every person needs to revisit or aspire to. We have been led to believe that young = desirable, so as women age, we become less desirable. Why else are magic formula face creams so popular, a tool for women to turn the clock back and erase the wrinkles written on our bodies? Erasing the record of our lives with an elixir for eternal youth. If only the Knights Templar could have gone to the chemists for a lotion or potion! On a more disturbing level, it is clear that patriarchy reveres the Maiden at the expense of her innocence and wellbeing. Pornography involving actual underage teenage girls is some of the most viewed online porn. Pornography providers such as Pornhub have further victimised underage girls by failing to recognise these images as abuse and, therefore, illegal, meaning that there are abusers who need to be found and prosecuted. Sites like Pornhub, Youporn and Mydirtyhabit have all knowingly exploited children for profit, profits that come from the abuse and unlawful sexualisation of the young. Hopefully, Pornhub is on its last grubby legs. At the time of my writing, thanks to the Justice Defence Fund, the business is facing lawsuits which seek to prosecute the providing of images of abused teenage girls, along with the unlawful images involving trafficked women. Germany seems set to be one of the first countries to shut down Pornhub. Patriarchy's dangerous obsession with virginity is blatantly demonstrated by patriarchal regimes, like Yemen's Huthi regime, which enforces virginity testing on female prisoners and detainees. Virginity testing is an act of sexual violence. Thank Goddess for Human Rights pressure groups who work to stamp out these abhorrent acts against women. According to Amnesty, women in Yemen face 'rampant discrimination and are subjected to highly conservative cultural gender norms'.[6]

Mother

The Maiden falls from patriarchy's pedestal when she receives her bleed and enters the cycle of Mother. This is blood that patriarchy wants to hide and shame. Many male-penned religious doctrines view menstrual blood as unclean, making the woman unclean for this part of her cycle or, under some fundamentalist religious interpretations, unclean simply for being a woman. The upside-down logic here is that women need a menstrual cycle to naturally produce the young which patriarchy feels entitled to plant within our bodies. The world needs the menstrual cycle to create new life but patriarchy shames its existence. When the woman is in her years of bleeding, she is shamed for her cycle because her blood makes her too much. In other words, if we are to honour the true power of her blood, she is, in fact, too powerful, too mysterious, too magic, too earthy, and too intuitive for patriarchy to bear.

Wise Woman

The next cycle of the woman's life sees the unfolding of the menopause and the eventual cease of her blood. Her blood stays inside and the menstrual cycle stops. During this process, the woman enters the realm of the Wise Woman. She may feel a deeper connection with the lunar phases or start tuning into moon magic to mark the ebbs and flows of her life. The relationship between women and the moon is an ancient one. Pagans have been marking the flow of the moon phases for thousands of years, and witches gather at the dark moon to thank the Great Goddess for her help with manifesting magic on Earth. Unsurprisingly, patriarchal society does not hold the menopause and ageing process in any esteem. Under the patriarchal lens, when women lose their menstrual cycle and the potential to be baby machines, which men feel entitled to use to incubate their sperm, they fall once again. The ageing woman seems not to deserve respect, much less be seen as desirable, because she is no longer fertile. For patriarchy, she no longer has the use of child-bearing; *Quick, get one of Margaret Atwood's Handmaids on speed dial!* Interestingly, I hear from my older woman friends that their menopause was the time when they felt authentically able to give zero fucks about societal BS, seeing through the veil of fuckery, feeling able to say and act as they please. A timely response for how society views female ageing and menopause! My thoughts turn to the treatment of women in Eastern countries like Iran, Saudi Arabia, and Yemen who are not afforded the same freedoms as women in the West to express a zero fucks attitude. Yes, women are too much for state-sanctioned patriarchy. Too much and proud. What if as we age, we all aspire to be the kind of too much that patriarchy shames? The kind that feels our feelings, asking for what we want and saying no to what we don't want, dressing however we like, witnessing and honouring our ageing process, allowing our bodies to change and choosing exercise and foods which support our cycles?

I believe I am right in guessing that the menstrual cycle, female ageing and menopause are not hot topics of male conversation, whether it be with their female partner or with their blokes down the pub. There are anomalies, though, men who are comfortable discussing these super important topics, ones who want to educate themselves about how they can support their female partner as she cycles through her life cycles. My boyfriend is one of these chaps who has become more comfortable hearing about blood, ageing, patriarchy, and menopause. I have led by example, though, and refused to censor myself on these crucial chats because I used to be with a man who winced at the sight of a tampon and thought a scheme should exist to gene-test girlfriends to predict how well they may age and check that they had no defects to pass on to future children. Eugenics is not dead. Generally, it's like patriarchy wants to pretend that ageing, cycles, and bleeding do not happen. Similarly, women have been taught to hide the flow of their blood by using tampons pre-menopause and taking HRT to keep young during menopause. I bet if men had to stick a piece of cotton inside their genitals to soak up blood, we would never hear the end of it.

Patriarchy picks and chooses when ageing and the menstrual cycle are in favour. They want to de-cherry young women and make girls sexually active, then they feel grossed out by periods, unwilling to support the emotional needs of a woman in her menstrual cycle, then they want us in good condition and ovulating nicely so they can knock us up, then they want us to hide our menstrual cycle from them when babies are not on the to-do list, but then they miss it when the menstrual is swapped for the magic of the menopause. They do not want to ejaculate their precious seed on to non-fertile land. When it comes to bleeding, women are, again, damned if we do and damned if we don't.

Crone

When women reach much later life and enter into the cycle of the Crone, this is the cycle that patriarchy does its damndest to conceal. If you grew up in amongst a white, patriarchal, capitalist society, you will realise that this society worships beauty and youth while hides old age. The Crone is the most challenging female archetype because she is at an age where she is closer to death than the Maiden, Mother or Wise Woman. She represents decay, destruction, and death, which are all part of the bigger life cycle. There is a Celtic Goddess called Sheela na Gig, who is the ultimate embodiment of the Crone. She is old, wizened and depicted on sacred sites with her vagina on show for all to see. Traditionally the Crone was the teacher of the seers, medicine women and midwives. She would bestow her knowledge of the cycle of life, the process of life, death, and life again. She held firm to her wisdom that the decay before death is not simply the end. Rather, this is the time when the earthly body decays while the soul or spirit gets closer to returning to the Source/Universe/Creator. The dead body decays into the Earth or the sea, or the ashes are scattered onto the land to become part of the ongoing ecosystem which gives life to the plants, mammals, fish and creepy crawlers.

Patriarchy has tried to manipulate people into believing that the elders, particularly the women elders, have no use. They either make her invisible or portray her as a burden, an embarrassment who is obsolete to the onward march of youth-focused technocratic society. What could the Crone possibly have to offer in this world which moves fast and takes no prisoners? The world, which is presided over by government with a penchant for technocracy, bit by bit is marginalising its elders. It both breaks my heart and boils my blood when life is made difficult for our elders. Not all old people have smartphones for apps to listen to what used to be the radio, not all old people have access to or want to use the internet, not all old people have debit cards or apps to tap to pay for goods while the West tiptoes toward a cashless society (cashless means increased surveillance of our habits and movements). The UK government showed its utter disdain for society's elders by shoving Covid patients into old folks' homes and letting the virus run riot in these so-called care homes. This was an orchestrated cull of the elderly, the ones whom the system deems surplus to requirements. That is what the government think of our grandparents. Their actions during the Coronavirus outbreak speak far louder than any political rhetoric about protecting the elderly and vulnerable, oozing from the mouths of the identikit-suited and booted Westminster elite. In May 2020, my 90-year-old great uncle Ron was paid a home visit by an NHS worker to ask him to sign a 'Do Not Resuscitate' agreement should he get hospitalised with Covid. The admin worker showed up on his property because my uncle had not responded to their previous letter asking his consent for DNR. Uncle Ron sent her packing from his doorstep, refusing his consent and form unsigned, professing that there was life in this old dog yet. I was bursting with pride that he stood up for his right to live when faced with such an evil agenda.

What the Crone has for the world is decades of blood wisdom from her periods, decades of wisdom for how to navigate patriarchy, decades of experience from raising her own children or the wisdom she gained from reparenting herself, decades of the knowledge of love and loss. Perhaps most importantly, she symbolises wisdom of one for whom death is not so far away. Her power and wisdom are too much for the system to bear! The Crone's power and wisdom were reduced to the lurid, cartoony images of warty witches and decrepit old hags thanks to Church propaganda in medieval Europe. The Church suppressed the possibility that life is a cycle in which our dead bodies feed the Earth because they wanted to firmly sever the link between people and nature, particularly women and nature. If women understood (as many of us already understand and many of us are remembering) that they were part of the Earth, rather than put on the Earth by God as per biblical stories, it would be a damn sight harder for the Church to control women, when it set the patriarchal ball rolling so long ago. These days it seems as if society does not want to see the Crone because the reminder of approaching death is unpalatable. Western society hides from death and pathologises grief as if death can never be accepted as part of our life cycle. Patriarchy reveres the strongest and fittest, the healthiest, the lithe and youthful.

We have seen the outcome of these preferences before under Naziism and totalitarian regimes. It never ends well. The system craves an elixir for eternal youth, which is nowhere to be seen in the body of an old, bowed, wrinkled woman who has spent life under the insidious oppression of patriarchy.

I think Crones are the fucking best. One of my grandmothers is in her nineties and has severe memory loss, but she does what she can, and I feel amazed every day that she is still here. My other grandmother died in her 90s in 2022. Both of these women, both called Gwendoline, looked after me when I was very small when my mum had to return to work. My maternal gran would make me fish fingers, mashed potatoes and tinned tomatoes for lunch, while Nan from my dad's side of the family preferred to treat me to Billy Bear and ketchup sandwiches. If you are not familiar with Billy Bear, look him up. I don't eat this yummily nostalgic food now because I'm vegan, but the sight of this odd luncheon meat still fills me with joy! I used to play behind the fir trees at the top of Gran's garden and look for fossils among the gravel. She did not seem to get bored of me showing her random bits of non-fossils that I found. When I went to Nan's, we would walk around town window shopping and usually bump into elderly people that she and Grandad had known for years. To me, these people were elderly, but to my grandparents, they were just people who had stories to tell and memories to reminisce on. To my three-year-old self, it was like everybody in Gloucester knew Nan and Grandad. I was proud to walk around with them. My grandmothers taught me that 'old age does not come alone'. They were referring to the ailments, body changes, and forgetfulness that were making their way into their lives, but I like to think that the other visitor with old age is wisdom.

Whether our bodies are cycling through Maiden, Mother, Wise Woman, or Crone, we can lean into our wisdom to deconstruct the conditioning that we need our bodies to be anything that patriarchy dictates.

Women have differing bodies, so back off let women get on with it is what I say. Young or old, bleeding or menopausal, fat or thin, abled or with a disability, we have always been enough. More than enough. I pray that women will continue to lift up their voices to speak out about the diseases and conditions that patriarchy does not want to know about.

Rising

What do you want to tell your younger self about the ageing process? Write a letter to her.

Which cycle are you feeling most resonant with: Maiden, Mother, Wise Woman, or Crone? Or perhaps a blend of them all?

What messaging did you receive about the female body while you were growing up? Consider the words and actions of caregivers, elders, friends, media, religion, and schooling.

What is your body to you? A place of power or conflict? Something to flow with or something to control? There are no 'right' answers here. Be real.

If you could choose to (because you can), what would you choose to believe and feel about your body?

Visualise or look in the mirror at your unmade-up, unshaven, unwashed, naked (if that is comfortable for you) body. In your opinion, is She too much or not enough or both? Acceptable or damn delicious?

There has been a surge in the popularity of the body positivity movement in recent years. What are your feelings about this?

Do you have a disability? How much do you think the body positivity movement represents disability?

Do you feel able to maintain autonomy over your body?

Create a gorgeous collage to celebrate your current life cycle, Maiden, Mother, Wise Woman, or Crone, or combine all of them.

Talking of bodies, I hope you don't get queasy because our next chapter is about blood.

Lines on our bodies like layers of a rose.

A blood red rose.

Nature's palimpsest.

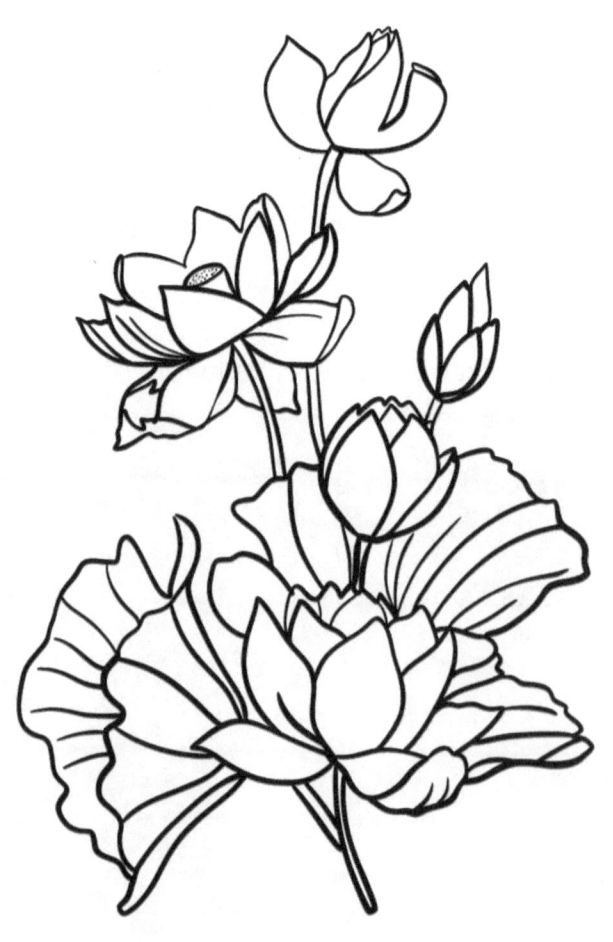

CHAPTER TEN

Blood

Rest

Make your way over to the Enough! area of my website and settle in for your deep rest practice where we will soften and release the lower body.

Recovery

> 'I just don't trust anything that
> bleeds for five days and doesn't die.'
> – Mr Garrison, South Park

What immediately comes to mind or to your heart when you think about your menstrual cycle? If you are not having periods or you are in menopause, you still have a cycle, so ask yourself, what have you been taught about the cyclic nature of the female body and the cycles you feel unfolding for you? What did your upbringing show you about cycles and periods?

Patriarchy is not a friendly place for your period. There is so much BS out there about what bleeding means about women and so much of this BS fuels the curse of too much and not enough. For aeons, women have been alluded to by males as unpredictable, hysterical, irrational, illogical, mysterious and not in a good way because of the cyclic nature of how we roll physically, emotionally, and mentally. Women are not supposed to feel the same every damn day simply due to highly nuanced and fluctuating levels of hormones being secreted, absorbed, and disposed of by our endocrine system. The varying levels of oestrogen, progesterone, testosterone, follicle-stimulating hormone and luteinising hormone all collaborate to support us through each cycle of approximately 28 days. Let me also be real and say that I am aware that many women do not have a cycle of the normalised 28 days, and that I am aware that an out-of-whack cycle can be a fucking nightmare rather than an enjoyable monthly process. If you are having difficulty with your cycle, be it anything from endometriosis to anxiety, please look up the period-tastic work of Alisa Vitti. Alisa is a female health specialist with over thirty years of experience when it comes to studying the menstrual hormones. Her book *In the FLO* helped me heal my pre-menstrual and menstrual depression.

Ok, back to the hormones. These carefully evolved and designed hormonal levels, which dance in a mind-boggling choreographed fashion, are the backdrop to the way we feel from week to week each menstrual cycle. Hormones influence our moods, behaviour, energy levels, food intake, sex drive, concentration levels and general mojo during each mini-cycle of the full menstrual cycle. I wish I had been told this nugget of information back in high school. What I am saying here about hormones does not even scratch the surface, but the point I am making is that women are not designed to feel the same, act the same, relate to people the same or even be interested in the same things at each part of the monthly cycle. Do not get me wrong, there are many things that we are capable of at any time of our menstrual cycle, but just because we can does not mean that pulling all-nighters, getting totally pissed, working 12-hour days, and rollerblading in white lycra while bleeding is supportive to the intricate work that the body needs to do during each part of the cycle. The more we try to do the busy or productive thing on the daily, the more tired and wired we are likely to become, which may lead to hormone imbalances during next month's cycle. Our hormones simply do not allow us to sustain the same consistently high levels of productivity, patience, compassion, kindness, badassery, holding-shit-together-ness, organisation, confidence, creativity, focused attention, perfect-in-every-way-ness, 'lady in the street but a freak in the bed' (which RnB singer Usher longs for in his track 'Yeah') that patriarchy demands from us.

The Pain is Real

Thousands of us suffer from hormone related menstrual conditions such as polycystic ovary syndrome, endometriosis, fibroids, PMDD (pre-menstrual dysphoric disorder), and menstrual depression, to name but a few. These genuine medical complaints mean that women are frequently trying to cope with anything from periodic to chronic pain. The system does not give us much leeway when we face this pain. We must either push through to stay productive because workplaces usually do not like to let women take time off to rest so that symptoms might ease. Or we are so debilitated that only strong painkillers, hot water bottles, and bed will help (this was often the case for me). Or the GP will prescribe the pill to stop the natural release of hormones to remedy the painful symptoms of the menstrual cycle. There is absolutely nothing wrong with women choosing the pill to get some relief from menstrual symptoms. What is problematic from the context of a patriarchal medical establishment model is that the menstrual cycle is not the domain of general practitioners because it is under-researched and not explored in minute detail in medical school, while menstrual cycle issues have a tendency to be disregarded as being all in the woman's head. It is unusual for family doctors to guide a woman through a hormone balancing protocol designed to support the body with easing symptoms using a non-synthetic approach. The usual options for hormone-related menstrual discomfort are put up, shut up, suppress it, ignore it, push through it, and be overly quick to medicate it. If you are one of the thousands of women who suffer from menstrual or hormone-related conditions, do seek help because you deserve better than to keep suffering. See what your doctor has to say if you feel able to discuss this with them, and I absolutely recommend reading the work of Alisa Vitti and her method for balancing hormones, along with the excellent guide to the menstrual cycle called *Code Red* by Lisa Lister.

Periods are cast as unproductive for women who have soaked up the myth that to be useful, accepted, or enough, we must be on our A-game all day, every day. The fallacy that women are hard to relate with, ailing, inconvenient bleeders who have no rhyme or reason to our monthly ups and downs, reinforces patriarchy's disdain for the female cycles. Trying to work around the pain of these conditions to live our best (e.g., being good enough) life at all times only exacerbates hormone imbalances, which worsen the symptoms of the myriad conditions that women are faced with navigating every month.

Patriarchy peddles the myth that we are too much because of the many physical and emotional changes we cycle through each month. Yet if we stop for an hour or so to do nothing but rest when we bleed, we are viewed as somehow defective and we risk the many plates we spin to come crashing down. In rest workshops I have held, when women discuss commonly held beliefs about their menstrual cycles and rest, there is a common concern that the bottom will fall out of every aspect of life should she take some time off from family-work-fitness-lover-spouse-partner-house labour duty (yep, even just 30 minutes).

There is also the overarching belief that they are selfish for daring to take time for themselves. Selfishness has its place. If more women were self-focused and taking proper bleed time for themselves, imagine the benefits to society as a whole. I have a friend who wants to make a community bleed space for women. Yes, please! I believe we got here because we were taught that we are bad/weird/flawed/inconvenient because we bleed and therefore must compensate for it.

Boy Talk

Boys were shielded from learning about periods when I was in school. I remember so vividly one of the very few lessons in school which attempted to teach about puberty and periods. There was one lesson as part of personal and social education and one lesson as part of the science curriculum for the age 13-14 group, which was repeated in a little more detail when it came time to study for the supposedly all-important GCSE exams the following year. In the PSE lesson, the boys were taken to a different room with a male teacher while the girls stayed in the form room with our female teacher. The girls learned about what to expect when our periods came: some bleeding from the vagina for a few days, which we should soak up with a sanitary towel or, preferably, a tampon because tampons would be more discreet, not visible as an outline under the tiny gym shorts which were regulation uniform for sports. (Honestly, these shorts were like the smallest hot pants which left nothing to the imagination. Looking back, it doesn't seem totes appropes for teen girls to be running around in these, watched over by male gym teachers, some only about ten years older than us.) We were also reliably informed that tampons would mean we would not have to skip swimming because the blood would be held inside our bodies and would not dirty the water if we wanted to swim on our periods. Clearly, it is not hygienic to have menstrual blood leaking into swimming pools, but the emphasis was on the idea that it would be unpleasant for us and other people to see the blood at any point. The use of the word 'dirty' speaks for itself. Dirty blood equals dirty woman who needs to keep her blood out of sight lest it offend anybody. My school did not deem it necessary for the boys to learn about periods and menstrual products, and the girls did not need to learn about wet dreams and erections. And people wonder why men and women often struggle to communicate with each other, not least about sex and the menstrual cycle. It seemed like these topics were too much, too taboo, too irrelevant to the respective gender groups to be taught in the same classroom. This perpetuates the premise that men and women cannot ever really understand each other while the results of puberty are on a strictly need-to-know basis based on what genitalia one has.

Growing up, I only ever saw boys and later men be on a sliding scale of anything from squeamish about periods to full-on misogynist about bleeding (a boy in my school wrote a note to a girlfriend of mine saying he wanted to fuck her so hard until she bled 'worse' than on her period). In my twenties, a boyfriend told me that he didn't want to have sex with me when I was bleeding on my break from the pill because his 'dick did not look good with period on it'. I told myself that the blood meant I was not good enough for him, undesirable. I look back now and wonder if he felt that the blood was too much, too female to meet his penis that he was clearly so proud of. Maybe joint lessons about puberty would have normalised the physicality of the menstrual cycle, breaking away from the fallacy that these are only women's issues and hormone-related things are women's problems, much less that the menstrual cycle and the ongoing shifts in the female landscape are something to be honoured by all. In the same way, group teaching about erectile function may have dispelled the myth that if a bloke cannot get an erection, it must be because the prospective sexual partner is not attractive enough.

Blood Arrival

I got my first period in the changing rooms at Tammy Girl at age 11. I was trying on a long floaty lilac skirt with a print like violet waves and a white crop top. I wanted to wear it for the school disco. I looked in the long mirror and thought this outfit choice was exactly right. The skirt completely covered my legs which, ages ago, I decided were fat so they must never see the light from about the knee upwards. The strappy top showed off my belly button, which is what all the girls from school were wearing, and the straps meant that my bra straps were visible, which signalled to my peers, *I am terribly mature and practically a grown up because I need to wear a bra now.* This was a confusing time for me because my eleven-year-old self wanted to fit in with the girls at school who all wore eyeliner, silver hoops, and crop tops. Everybody was dressing older than their age because that is what we wanted: to assert ourselves as no longer children but have zero responsibility of teenagers with the mounting piles of homework and pressure to think about your future at every step. My school conditioned us young ones to be obsessed with trying to figure out our futures by choosing the right friends, the right behaviour, the right exam subjects, the right volunteering gig because it will look good on the CV. (Yep, seriously, at age 11 we were being spoken to about CVs to help show us off/prove we were enough to warrant that coveted uni place and that coveted job in that competitive career.) Just writing about those school years makes me feel uneasy and a little sweaty, remembering the constantly creeping anxiety that everything needed to be just right so as not to mess up your future.

Back to my disco outfit in the Tammy Girl changing rooms. I looked in the mirror and liked what I saw. This was very rare. I turned away from the mirror to get back into my other clothes when I felt it. I suddenly felt very hot and damp between my legs. I was convinced I had wet myself. My mind raced, trying to find a solution to wetting myself in my knickers in a busy shop on a Saturday which was packed with other eleven-year-olds all queuing to try on their own disco outfits. When I dared to look down, seeing that bright, cherry-red, thick pool in my knickers, it was as if time stopped. I was bleeding. I knew what was happening and this was not the place where I wanted to get my first period. My face flushed red and I started to sweat. What was I meant to do now? It was lucky that the skirt fitted and I liked it because there was a little blood on the inside of the material. Bright red daubed on the lilac canvas like a piece of modern art. I felt scared. Mainly because I needed to get this outfit paid for immediately by Dad, who was patiently waiting in the shop, pray that the cashier would not notice my blood on the skirt, and then scuttle off to the arcade toilets, a heady mix of potentially embarrassing scenarios ready to shame me in the middle of a busy Saturday shopping trip. There was more fear underneath this. Seeing my blood frightened me. There was something primal and fierce about the blood in my knickers which my eyes were fixed on. I did not feel ready for this and wished that could scrub it out, go back to being my eleven-year-old self playing at being a grown-up in my floaty skirt and crop top. Something had changed, like I did not know myself anymore, and truly that felt weirdly exciting in my heart while I was being given a glimpse of a part of life that I knew nothing about. I knew what my science textbooks said; *each month that the egg is not fertilised, it will be released and this is a woman's period.* Even at age eleven, I knew that there was waaaaaay more to this period business than some blood coming out of my girl parts (I winced at the word vagina at age eleven!). It was all intuition and I had no facts to go on, but I knew I was changed forever. I was initiated into being a woman by my blood in a shop for girls. Cosmic signposting.

Skirt paid for, I made an excuse and dashed off to the shopping arcade toilets. There was a big coffee shop downstairs from the loos, and as I dashed across the mezzanine, my nostrils feasted on the smell of pastries, the cups and saucers clinked, the murmur of shoppers and the noise of the coffee machine's milk frothing travelled upstairs. I was tunnel visioned, I needed to get to the cubicle! Cubicle reached, I locked myself in the loo, hands quivering at the lock. I grabbed a handful of loo roll and stuffed it into my knickers, my first foray into the world of sanitary wear.

When I got home, somehow, my mum had guessed that I was having a period, either that or my dad guessed and told her. Mum took me upstairs to her room and opened her wardrobe. I thought wardrobes were exciting places thanks to C.S Lewis' book *The Lion, the Witch and the Wardrobe*, so I was absolutely ready for the wardrobe portal to open to show me a world I had never seen before. In some ways, this is what happened. My mum delved to the back and fished out a bag of sanitary towels. She had been so sweetly keeping this for me for a while and now I would need to use one every time I bled. She showed me how to put one into my knickers and told me periods were part of the curse of being a woman. She was only half joking. *Oh shit*, I thought, *this is seriously bad news*. Mum snaffled the sanitary towels into the back of the bathroom cabinet, gave me a hug, and we got on with our day. Is this where bleeding belonged? Shoved into a cupboard, out of sight, out of mind.

We need to celebrate the first bleed, show it off, or at the very least, tell our girls it is nothing to worry about. Imagine if that was a normal thing to do. I was sure it wouldn't matter if we just kept the Bodyform packet on the shelf where we could see it, but at age 11, I never questioned it. Hiding the period products speaks to the fact that society does not want to see our menstrual blood. The blood is too much simply because it releases from the female body, which religion made sure thousands of years ago was known as the epitome of unclean. The consensus across modern religion and secular thought is that men do not want to see women when we are menstruating – and forget about actually seeing our blood. In some denominations of Orthodox Christianity and Orthodox Judaism, women are not permitted to enter holy buildings or associate with men at the time of menstruation as 'not even they themselves, being faithful and pious, would dare when in this state either to approach the Holy Table or to touch the body and blood of Christ'.[1] The Quran labels menstrual blood as haram (forbidden), and so men must 'stay away from women during menstruation' (Al-Quran 2:222-223). For the record, I do believe that women need a break from men folk at bleed time, but not because we are supposedly unclean!

Cycle Love

I don't have religious beliefs, and I don't particularly feel like being around men when I get my period, preferring to chill with women or be on my own curled up in my duvet with my journal and pen. I also do not enter many religious buildings, I prefer to think of my own body as a sacred site instead of needing to go somewhere labelled as holy by patriarchal religions. What is problematic, though, about these very old-school religious views is that choice was taken from women, and their movements when menstruating were decreed by religious patriarchal doctrines, which, you guessed it, were penned by men. Women's autonomy was stolen in favour of pleasing the male God, keeping the offensive blood away from him. What doesn't make sense to me is that if God is supposedly loving and forgiving, would he be upset by a bit of blood? Of course not. But confusing paradoxes are all part of the patriarchal plan to reinforce the labelling of Femininity as both too much and not enough.

It's not just religion that wants to keep menstrual blood in the shadows. Artists who are inspired by menstruation and also who work in the medium of menstrual blood have been censored from Instagram.

It's fucked up, isn't it, that social media is a platform where girls are bullied into sending nude selfies way before they are ready to experience their sexuality, where women feel pressured to post the perfect pregnancy shots, where men get to toast their #Dadgoals and #Dadbods but art about the menstrual cycle, so fundamental to every human's life, was deemed inappropriate for public consumption.

Rising

Consider your own cycle (menstrual or not). Is there a time of the month when you feel at your most alive?

What are the cyclical recurring events in your life that trigger feelings of being not enough or too much?

What did your upbringing show you about cycles and periods?

Do you feel at home comparing period notes with your friends?

If you could celebrate your first period, how would you mark the occasion? Go and enjoy doing that.

If you fancy some movement, check out my yoga for the sacral chakra video on my website under the Enough! section.

I always related to my body as a minefield of too much and not enough, me and every other woman who grew up inside patriarchal conditioning! But when we bring somebody else's body into the mix, somebody we might fancy having sex with, that is when patriarchy's curse of too much and not enough gets even louder. Let's talk about fucking.

A force of nature lives inside you

From your cells to your atoms

Let it unravel

Feel it rise and flow

No more binding

Take up the space

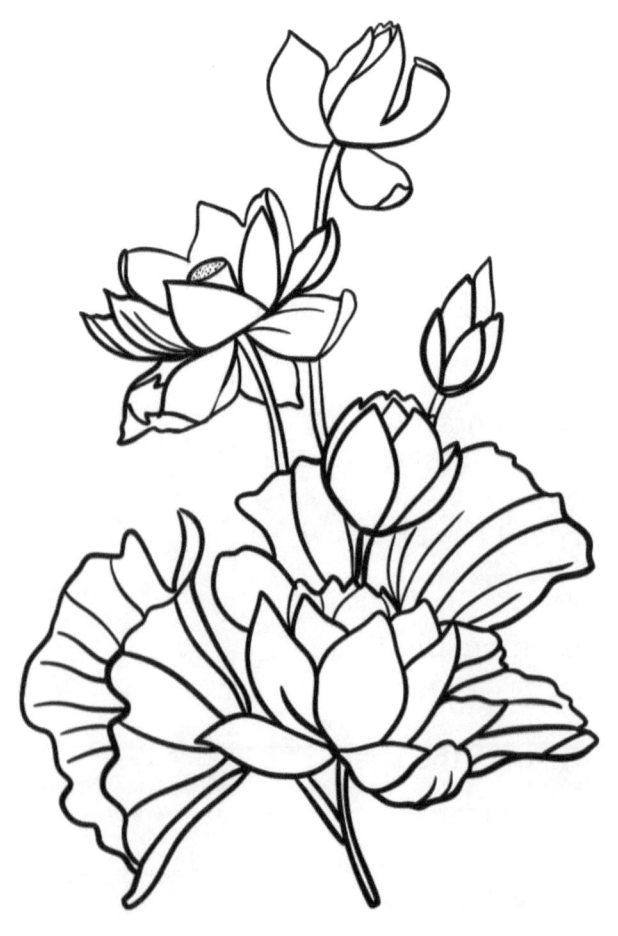

CHAPTER ELEVEN

Fucking

Rest

For this chapter, we let the earth hold us in our resting meditation.

Recovery

I would bet big money that all women have a tale to tell about sex. The good sex, the bad sex, the what-was-I-thinking sex, the this-is-so-much-more-than-just-sex sex, the drunk sex, the sober sex, the we-should-not-be-doing-this sex, the I-am-going-to-marry-him/her/them sex, the just-one-last-time sex, the so-hard-and-so-often-that-I-got-cystitis sex. There are a lot of things that can lead us to feel pretty unsexy about having sex. While growing up (and I class growing up as before age thirty), the messaging that

I soaked in regarding sex was that it was something for the guys to enjoy. Thank you, patriarchy, for this absolute fucker of a myth. Remember the boys I wrote about from my school? As well as talking about who has the best tits, as we got older, they would ponder about the girls' bedroom abilities, as if they were speculating about the fictional sex resume' of particular girls in our year. It went something like this:

> Boy A: Do you reckon she does (fill in the blank with any sex act here)?
>
> Boy B: Yeah, I reckon she (add a comment about how much she enjoys said sex act).
>
> Boy A: Oi (insert a girl's name here), Jack says you give (insert sex act). Is that true?

Boys will be boys, huh?

It was my turn to be the subject of this sexual baiting. Aged 15, I was at a party where all the Year 10s could illegally be served with cheap alcohol. A few Archers and lemonades down, I enjoyed some very public dancefloor and sofa-based snogs with an eligible boy in my year. Not going to lie, I loved it. I loved his hands in my hair, the aroma of Tommy Hilfiger on his chest and the little wet patch forming in my knickers. I hoped I was doing it right because I'd learned by 15 that boys liked girls who were up for it, and I wanted him to like me. It would be a signal for my very low self-esteem that all was not lost because I could get boys to like me by being good at snogging. I had fancied him for ages, and he had signalled for a few days in that adorable teenage way that he thought I was alright too. He used to put his arm round me to walk between classes and I thought I might spontaneously combust. I was keen to delay my combustion until I had at least found some way to dredge up the courage to tell him I liked him. How the fuck I was going to confess my teenage love for him, I had no idea because I was shit scared of getting turned down, and even worse than the almost certain rejection would be the whole of Year 10 knowing I was not good enough. Social suicide. So I never told him I liked him. I waited for the party, safe in the knowledge that I could get drunk. Hopefully, he would be drunk too so that the magic would happen when we fell into each other's arms and he would ask me out.

We snogged a lot that night. He never asked me out. Instead, on Monday, one of his mates bowled up to me and announced:

'Tom says you take it up the arse.'

'What?! No! That never happened!'

'Everyone's sayin' you did it in the rugby club toilets.'

'That's not true.'

'Don't blame me, I'm just sayin' what everyone's been sayin'.'

Most of our mates were indeed sayin' this dalliance had happened.

Me: 'Why are you saying this?'

Tom: 'I didn't. It's just a someone having a laugh.'

It turned out that Tom had not made up this story, but one of his mates had conjured up the rumour for all of Year 10 to enjoy. Everyone except me. The hero of the tale was getting a ton of macho praise, joking with his mates about supposedly fucking me. Me, I was awarded with dirty looks, whispering, side eyes, and:

'Oh my God, how could you let him do that? It's gross!'

Winners and Losers

I was confused, but soon it all became clear. Even if I had, in fact, done what was being said about me, in social terms and thanks to patriarchy which I had never heard of aged 15, Tom would have still been the winner. Even in the hypothetical situation of a high school rumour, the person in possession of the power to enjoy this fictional fuck was the man. As the female, I had served what was apparently my purpose of being a receptacle for his penis, only to be shit-talked about after. Any enjoyment of our non-existent sex seemed to be reserved for him.

I ruminated. *How come this rumour started anyway?* I rolled the question around my brain. I lost sleep over it. It did not seem fair. There I was, enjoying my snog with the object of my teenage affections, feeling like I was glistening in fairy dust from the inside out. For a few minutes, all was right with my world. When I used to snog boys, Tom included, I knew that I could feel something. This something felt electric, thrilling, filling my body with pulsating tingles. My heart would also feel seen, as if my heart and his were creating something very right, natural and beautiful. But then I end up getting the piss taken out of me, being the butt of somebody's joke, and Tom wouldn't even kill off the rumour by telling our mates it was not true. *I probably shouldn't have looked like I was enjoying myself so much, maybe I gave people the wrong idea about me? I should try not to feel those things.* I was confused again. My confused conclusion was as follows: I needed to look like I was having a good time in any future snogs (or sex when I could finally cut my virginity loose) to make sure the dude felt like things were going well, but I must not connect too much with myself to feel my own enjoyment and ignore the inevitable oxytocin release, because somebody might notice, and I will look like I'm having too much of a good time, not leaving enough room for the man's enjoyment. If I enjoyed myself *for* myself, was I being too much? The myth was playing out: I was Lilith and now I was being ostracised.

Jesus. No wonder I was confused about boys and sex; a woman is not enough if she does not appear to be turned on and sexy, but she is too much for even having, let alone following the feelings so naturally produced by the female body just doing its thing during snogging and sex. I had inadvertently objectified myself and bought into the patriarchal conditioning, which I would later explore in school when I met *The Handmaid's Tale* in English Lit class. At age 15, I could not see that I had already become a part of the conditioning. The world was not showing me anything different. Sex was one for the boys, forget about a woman being free to actually properly enjoy herself. The first time I had sex, I was terrified of looking like I was getting it wrong by letting myself feel it. It was an awkward encounter. I was glad that it barely lasted two minutes. I was also scared to move my body in case he saw what I perceived were my fat thighs, fat bum, and fat stomach. I whispered to him as he started:

'Please don't look at my legs.'

Sex Skillset

I was a teen with body dysmorphia, so I did not want him to see too much of my body because I felt I just could not compare with the glamour model posters on every inch of his bedroom walls. I was laying there surrounded by posters of Katie Price and Nell McAndrew with their supposedly perfect bodies, lips pouting and that dead, 'get me out of here look' behind their eyes. *You are not like us*, they seemed to say. *You never will be.* Thing is, no woman has to uphold those glamour model standards. I wish I could go back in time and tell my younger self. We got brainwashed by those images of what a woman is meant to look like. Frankly, I think teenage boys are brainwashed by highly sexualised images of glamour women too; it is patriarchy storming in uninvited and showing boys what they are supposed to desire, twisting their minds to think they should expect these sexy caricatures of women. It is not real and horribly unfair to influence young people this way. Thanks to being stared down by these posters each time I was in his bedroom, I was kept excruciatingly aware of patriarchy's sexual requirements from women:

- Be up for it but not too much because that would make me a slut.
- Strive for a toned, smooth body with perfect hair, perfect make up, tiny waist, massive boobs and no pubic hair. (I've never understood why men get fixated with wanting to see zero pubic hair on a woman. Is it because they want to fuck pre-pubescent girls? Vile.)
- Be ready to please a man but not to expect too much in return.
- Be a performer of sex at the drop of a hat but do not really, deeply feel it.
- Stay detached from emotions.
- Dead behind the eyes.

What I did feel the first time I had sex was enough to let me know that I definitely enjoyed it, but I also understood that the focus was never to be on me. The focus was on the service I was providing. I learned the formula: look good so he gets hard then it happens. 'The old in-out' soliloquised by Alex in *A Clockwork Orange*. I tried to pretend that I was cool about sex. This was what I thought 'cool about sex' was: always be willing to do it and pretend I didn't need to feel respected or require any emotional connection from a partner. I understood that for a woman, sex was to be performative yet emotionally passive.

Curse of the V Plates

Ah well, at least I had lost my virginity. When you look back at your time in Virginville, were you keen to stay there a while longer, or did you feel pressure to lose your V plates? Unsurprisingly, as a teenager I realised I was dammed if I did lose my virginity and dammed if I clung to it for dear life. Why? Teenage Sarah thought she had to have sex with her boyfriend to keep him interested, or else he would find some other girl to go out with and I really did not want that. I wanted to stay with him so that I could feel better about myself. Co-dependent, much?! He was my ticket to feeling whole, to feeling enough. I felt pressured both by the kudos I thought I would get from my peer group if I chose to be de-cherried, but also pressured by my own gnawing sense of insecurity that if I did not lose my V-plates, I would lose him too. After our awkward unsexy encounter, I was worried he would dump me because he would lose interest in me, plus now I was being called a slut. I thought I had fucked it up by fucking him.

Patriarchy plays its unfunny tricks when people lose their virginity. The curse of too much and not enough seeps in to deliver another mindfuck of a situation for young women. The familiar scenario of boys being slapped on the back, fist bumped, congratulated by their mates after their first time having sex. A bizarrely contrasting response waited for young girls losing their virginity. When my boyfriend's mates found out that we were having sex, he received his slap on the back and congratulations, but they sneered and laughed about me, saying I was 'easy'. The girls in my year could not win. If we did have sex for the first time with our boyfriends, then we were looked down on by the boys and taunted for having 'loose pussies', too much to fit the mould of a mythical pure, untouched Maiden. If a girl did not want to lose her virginity, she was bullied for being 'tight', frigid, not enough to satisfy the guy. Sadly, the microcosm of playground taunting was a training ground for navigating the double standards of society.

What did being cool about sex mean for you when you were growing up? Were there times in your teens (or even now) which led you to believe you were not enough or too much when it came to sex? Perhaps an answer comes to your mind or a feeling to your body right away, or would you like to take more time to ponder that question? Go for it if so. What would it be like to discuss the question with a trusted friend or a therapist? This is a tender topic so please go gently with yourself. It is so important that women open up to each other about the sex-based conditioning we may have received while growing up. We cannot help but carry these beliefs and patterns around with us, patterns which colour our relationship with ourselves, our bodies, our partners, our enjoyment of sex.

To me, being cool about sex meant that I always needed to be available for sex when my boyfriend wanted it. As a horny teenager with tons of hormones buzzing about, this was not such a problem for me because I was super attracted to the boyfriend whom I had sex with for my first time. But, thanks to my first sexual experiences like the drunk snogging incident I had, unbeknownst to me, I was well on my way to forming the belief that the blokes were the important, powerful ones and that pleasing them would gain me approval. It went deeper than approval, though. I wanted to believe that I mattered, and if I was giving pleasure to a guy during sex, then for that short amount of time, I mattered. *This is why blokes want women around, for sex.* I often thought to myself. *This is how to make sure I matter.* I made my willingness to have sex into a currency which bought me approval. It made me feel good enough, but good enough never lasted, the dead eyes of the poster women on his walls saw to that.

DTF (Down to Fuck)

When I was about 14, I heard from a girlfriend that there was this tablet you could take that would stop your periods to make sure you would not get pregnant. She was taking it, she told me, because it meant that she could always have sex with her boyfriend and he did not have to wear condoms anymore. While my friend and I ate lunch in the Year 11 area, my friend informed me that boys hate wearing condoms because they are a pain to put on, plus they stop them from feeling anything during sex. Her boyfriend had told her that. He was older than her by a few years and she had met him on holiday. I thought she was the height of sophistication. She and her bloke had done it a few times without a condom, she said, and luckily she had not got pregnant, but now she was 'on the pill' so they didn't have to worry about that anymore. I remember that moment when my stomach lurched while I sensed the nervous sweat on my back: *my boyfriend must hate wearing condoms too. What if he's not enjoying having sex with me?* I concluded that I was not fulfilling my duty of being a perfect girlfriend by requiring him to go through what must be the total annoyance of putting on a condom. *I am expecting too much from him if I want him to fiddle about with contraception. I am too much for him.* What to do about this? For a while, I did nothing. I was too terrified of getting pregnant to have unprotected sex, and I did not want to go to my GP to ask for this wonder pill which my friend had found because my doctor was my family doctor. What if he told my parents? I would die from the shame. The GP's wife knew my mum too, they were in the village choir together. Oh, and Tim Maclean in my year, his dad is a GP at the same surgery. Too many links back to me made it far too risky.

Now, when I feel into my teenage thought process about asking my doctor for the pill, I feel echoes of my teenage uneasiness about going to ask a male authority figure for a medication to stop me getting pregnant. This is the work of patriarchy which leads a woman to doubt if it is OK for her to ask for what she needs, the fear of being denied something because a man says no, along with the fear of being judged. This is an ancient visceral imprint left over from our female ancestors who were denied their voice and autonomy. Remember our witches.

A few months later, I was prescribed the contraceptive pill to help clear up my acne. It was a last resort treatment, my doctor said, because I had tried ALL the other stuff. Teenage Sarah could not believe her luck, no more acne and no more condoms and no nightmares about getting pregnant. Result! The boyfriend and I sacked off using condoms and he could not have been happier:

'I fucking hate wearing condoms, you just can't feel anything. Such a mood killer to put on. Bareback is much better.'

I made a decision about sex that day, about what men needed to stay satisfied, about what I needed to give them so I could cling on to any sexual kudos. Age fifteen, I decided that I would not come off the wonder pill ever, in case I subjected a man to wearing the dreaded Durex. I concluded that I would be ready to fuck whenever because I was on the pill, and in my limited fifteen-year-old understanding, I had the edge over women who were not on contraception, as if I was a product which needed a unique selling point to market. I believed I was not enough, not desirable without the pill. Age fifteen, I wondered if there were other girls who felt that they needed this drug to A) make them desirable, and B) make life easier for their boyfriends.

I stayed on the pill until I was thirty-four. I lived in the warped idea that I would be sexually useless, undesirable if I required my partners to wear a condom while I stayed a slave to the desires of patriarchy. Fifteen-year-old Sarah was ruining my sex life. I got chlamydia twice, and I am damn lucky that was all I got during my pill-enabled dicing with my sexual health, but to my inner fifteen-year-old who believed that she would be unwanted if she was not on the pill and able to have sex at the drop of a hat (or knickers), a couple of courses of antibiotics for odd infection were worth it. I have grieved and wept for my younger self who thought it was OK to treat myself and other people this way. Aged twenty-three I was, sitting on my bed after a trip to the GUM clinic, texting all my sexual partners within the previous six months to let them know I may have infected them with chlamydia. They weren't so sympathetic, and I can't say I blame them.

Have you ever insisted that a bloke wear a condom? What happened? I hope he was obliging about it. How did you feel about insisting? Empowered or sheepish? I hope it was the former. I believed I was not enough without the pill and too much if I insisted he use one. A guy told me once:

'I love that you're on the pill, I can fuck you whenever I want.'

So much is problematic about his statement, but back then, I totally agreed. I loved being able to have sex without worrying about getting preggers and no awkward vibe-ruining moments to find a condom. It suited me. I totally big up the pill and other methods of contraception for giving women sexual liberation to fuck who we want and whenever we want, because, let's be honest, who wants to be concerned about getting knocked up every time one has sex. The pill has also been a welcome stopgap from horrendous PMS and the body-shredding pain of periods for millions of women. Let's also thank Goddess for the morning-after pill and abortion clinics which save us from the trauma of unwanted pregnancies. Of course, there are religious fundamentalists who disagree with me about the matter of contraception and abortion, who believe that women who choose to protect against or terminate pregnancies should be sent one-way to the seventh circle of Hell for asking too much to have the right to choose what happens to their bodies. Whatever. I can do me, you do you. Thing is, I let myself be all about what I thought men wanted when it came to sex, pleasure, and contraception. The pearl of anti-condom wisdom from my friend, plus the opinion of my teenage boyfriend were fodder for the too much and not enough narrative; *do not be too much by asking too much of a bloke, e.g., to wear a condom because they 'fucking hate it', and without the edge of built-in contraception, you are not enough.* If I fucked somebody new, I would cringingly remind them to wear a condom. As I got older, this request came easier to me, but I never looked forward to that part. I did not see asking for contraception as the huge act of self-care that it truly is because I did not think I was worth it. Wait, it is not about being worth it because worth implies that there is a sliding scale of worthiness that says that some people are more worthy than others. We all have a right to protect our sexual health and protect against pregnancy (if we wish) in any safe way that we please.

In January 2019, I finished my last packet of oral contraceptive. I did not want the chemicals or the disconnection from my menstrual blood anymore. It was hard to override the habit of making the next doctor appointment to receive another prescription. I listened to my body and not my brain patterns on this one. For a long while, I was craving my menstrual cycle, the She inside me whom I had never gotten to know because of my long-term relationship with the pill. I wanted to know my cycle and four years on, we are still getting acquainted. I was proud and scared to announce to my boyfriend that I was coming off the pill so he would need to start wearing condoms. He was non-plussed:

'Of course,' he replied. Exhale. I felt my body soften. Liberation.

Pleasure and Play

How would you like to receive your pleasure? Perhaps this is an uncomfortable question for you. If it is not uncomfortable, perhaps it is a question that is unexplored. Women are anatomically designed to be receivers of pleasure. I loved reading in Regena Thomashauer's book *Pussy* that the entire point of the clitoris is to allow a woman to feel pleasure. There is literally no other reason for having this in-built pleasure receptor. This piece of clitoral wisdom was a game-changer for me in my late twenties. I learned that my body was a place to feel and receive pleasure, rather than a receptacle to be used for a bloke to get his rocks off. Sure, my vagina would feel pretty lovely during sex, but I had always believed that pleasure was kept mostly for the guys. I was definitely stuck believing that for us women, sex was meant to be performative rather than pleasurable; perform it, do not feel it, like the dead-behind-the-eyes glamour models who adorned teen boyfriend's bedroom walls. Any genuine flashes of sweet electricity felt in my body were not as important as the orgasm of my male partners, plus if I really let loose and felt what I was feeling right to my core, maybe something bad would happen. *Don't look like you're enjoying it too much, try not to feel those forbidden things, Sarah.* Maybe feeling pleasure would mean I was too much, and I would end up being cut loose from a partner for being an actual slut, instead of the pseudo-sluts my generation of guys seemed to crave. If I allowed myself to feel and follow my pleasure, would that mean that he was not getting his, or worse, was I depriving a woman elsewhere of getting pleasure?

Society teaches women that pleasure is a reward for previous effort. Remember those L'Oréal adverts from the 90s where Jennifer Aniston declared, 'You're worth it'? As if using Elvive shampoo and having the pleasure of shiny hair like Rachel from *Friends* should be seen as a reward for being worthy. Sorry, L'Oréal, but women are allowed to receive pleasure and have glossy hair whether they perceive themselves as worth it or not. You get to have pleasure just because. Fuck being worth it. It can feel scary to even admit that yes, we would like to feel pleasure, we can, in fact, feel pleasure and yes, we bloody well like it when we feel it. Of course, pleasure does not have to come from sexy time (alone or with a partner/s). Pleasure can be derived from truly savouring a yummy meal, twirling about to your favourite music, hanging out with a cherished friend, the warm sun or the aroma of fresh rain. When writing out that list, I just thought to myself, *Those things are all so delicious, does it really make sense to put them off?* Nope. I have tried to make my book-writing process something of a pleasure party. I seriously enjoy writing and adore plotting the rest practices that accompany the words, but it is also very definitely a type of work, albeit work which flows, and which feels purposeful, so there is pleasure which derives from the writing process itself. However, it is not me doing pleasure on purpose.

I purposefully seek out pleasure before working, which could be a long Yoga Nidrā practice, a dip in the sea, or simply taking the time to set up my writing space so it is inviting and beautiful, even just lighting a candle and wrapping myself in a blanket is enough. We do not have to look super far to receive a moment of pleasure. We may receive it from the scent of a rose, a piece of chocolate, the warmth of a long bath, the point is that we allow ourselves to have it. Just because.

Does asking for pleasure make us selfish? Nope. That nagging worry about being perceived as selfish is likely a learned neural code developed by watching the pleasure habits (or lack thereof) of our caregivers and role models as we grew up. If nobody demonstrated to you that it was necessary to receive pleasure to avoid spinning out into highly-strung neurosis, how the fuck were you supposed to learn and feel OK about getting your pleasure on? Does it mean that we will get out of control while listening to the body's need for enjoyment, nourishment, or fun rather than the logic of the brain with regard to how we should be spending our time? Pleasure versus work. Hmmm, which would we like to put first? What is the sensible choice? Sometimes it is OK to say: *Fuck Sensible. It's Pleasure Time!* (as long as *Fuck Sensible* means you or others are not being harmed). I do get it, though. *Fuck Sensible* doesn't always come easy.

Finding our pleasure as women is frowned upon by patriarchy. They would not want us pleasured up to our eyeballs the whole time because we would surely turn our back on our chores from childbearing to packed lunch packing. There is always something that needs our attention other than our pleasure. Thankfully, I don't have children to run around after, and I cannot imagine what it would be like to find the time to explore one's own pleasure away from the role of Mum. But women can do it, it is possible, and I admire the women around me who down tools to receive their pleasure in any way they damn well please. Perhaps they are such excellent mums because they do make space for their own enjoyment, so when they are called on to do the school run before working a demanding job until 6 pm and it is time to do baths and bedtime stories, they actually have enough fuel in the tank to take care of others because they have taken care of themselves. Again, pleasure needn't come from the overtly sexual. As a survivor of sexual violence myself, I know that exploring sexual pleasure can feel like a lot too soon. There is no need to override these feelings if it seems like sexual pleasure might overstep your current boundaries. Pleasure can come from the sensual too: a self-guided foot massage, the aroma that fills the kitchen when you make your favourite dish, getting lost in your armchair with the characters in a storybook. Topping up our sensuality reserves can start by playing with the idea of establishing a friendly relationship with your body, by moving in ways that feel good through dance and mindful movement, by getting quiet and feeling into the breath filling your belly, which literally inflates the sacral area in the low back and low belly. Do what feels good and right.

Witnessing Shame

What stops us from asking for and receiving our pleasure, whether this be derived from sex, lone sexy time, or indulging in dessert after dinner? Enter the well-known visitor called shame. Perhaps it is the shame of being labelled selfish for asking for what we want? Society shames women who dare put their needs above that of their families. We also have society to thank (or not!) for the echoes of shame that have trickled down to us from our ancestors, who were shamed for having beliefs that the church labelled as heresy. So much comes back to our witches who lived outside of patriarchal religious norms. There is sexual shame indoctrinated into women who simply want to feel their bodies, who know that pleasure has their name written all over it, from their pussies to their hearts and back again. We also cannot forget perhaps the most misplaced shame of all: shame triggered in a survivor of sexual violence. Survivors face the misplaced shame of being violated and the insidious, creeping doubt cast about by society that maybe, just maybe, they were partly responsible for what was done to them. *Perhaps the survivor was too drunk or too high or too provocatively dressed, perhaps they did not fight hard enough, perhaps they wanted it because they did not run away,* murmur the victim blamers. Well, shame can just fuck off.

My recovery from sexual violence has taught me about pleasure and shame. I have explored this topic more deeply in my first book, *Shadow & Rose*, to support other survivors on the recovery path. Shame cuts off the pathways to pleasure, but it is up to us to rewild those paths. While my therapist listened, I would ask my shame what it wanted me to know. Shame had a powerful message for me. This post-rape shame was not mine. I learned that I must not stay embroiled in the shame of what was done to me because the shame did not belong with me. It was shame which needed to be given back to the perpetrators. Shame on them for what they did. Shame on all the abusers who violate the sacred ground of another person's body and mind. Shame on the authorities who wilfully make it so hard to prosecute rape and sexual violence, which pretty much decriminalises abuse of women worldwide. I learned that my body was not the home of shame. Instead, I chose that my body would be a place of my own enjoyment. My body is a place where it is safe to feel the rising sensations of pleasure, they are mine to feel just because. I want this for all women, whether you happen to be a survivor of sexual violence or not. You reserve the right to your Feminine pleasure, whether it arises from sex or a scoop of your favourite ice cream.

I notice I feel I have not written enough about sex, pleasure, and patriarchy. I feel like I should have numerous more clever insights about this threesome of topics. Maybe the words on the page do not matter this time, maybe it is our own experiences and our own bodies which hold the key to our pleasure wisdom. Go explore. Give yourself full permission.

A Side Note: When Pleasure Is Not Pleasure

I will say it again, you are allowed to receive pleasure just because. Pleasure does not need to be put on the backburner for when you are less busy. Pleasure is not hard to access, look no further than the scent of your favourite flower or the joy that bubbles up when you connect with a treasured friend. These simple things provide accessible inroads to pleasure. The system we live in would have us believe that pleasure is scarce and hard to access, so one must cling on to and gobble up any tasty morsels of pleasure. Patriarchy not only wants you to believe that you are not enough, but also that there is not enough of any of the things that we might want, not enough money to go around, not enough food to go around, not enough work. The answer for this quandry? Seek out tons of things, pleasurable things, to make you feel better about yourself. Seek out things to provide relief from the system that drags you down, works you hard and leaves you feeling empty. Patriarchy combined with core beliefs about not being enough can trigger the endless search for things which provide pleasure as an escape both from the system and our own neurological systems, which fire thousands of thoughts a day around a familiar topic: not being enough. The searching for pleasure as an escape from the gaping hole of not enough is a foundation for addiction.

Addiction is not pleasurable but there are plenty of extremely pleasurable things to be addicted to. Choose a weapon for guaranteed self-destruction if you happen to be an addict. Let's begin with the obvious ones known for substance addiction: alcohol and drugs. Both of these offer the promise of pleasure, but the kind of pleasure which acts as an escape from oneself. I have had so much pleasure while on drugs, mainly Class As. There is not a day that goes by when I don't catch myself thinking about the ease of getting high, how much fun I had fuelled by heady concoctions of MDMA and cocaine. It used to be just on a weekend, then it was every weekend, and then cocaine was every day. The truth of it is that being high can be the most pleasure it is possible to imagine. One of the major tendencies for addiction is the unescapable foundational belief that you need external things to make your life better, more frankly, you need them to cope because, without them, you would implode down into the gaping hole of I-am-not-enough-ness. However, if you have no addictive tendencies, if you can handle the idea of never touching this substance/behaviour/person again, and you can hand on your heart say that this thing is not causing you harm, then crack on and enjoy an occasional dabble.

People can get high off the pleasure or escapism provided by loads of stuff; it does not need to be substances. It can be sex, relationships, work, social media, gaming, shopping, gambling, food, even the high of successfully being in control of one's body, as seen in eating disorders (yes, these are addictions). When you are seeking pleasure to satiate the grinding, gnawing emptiness that rules every waking minute, you will do anything to see to it that you get your fix of pleasure simply as a way of coping with life. Seeking out the thing is not pleasurable. I believed I would have no way of coping without the crutch of my eating disorder, and without the crutch of coke or the crutch of sex. We live in a world which coerces people to seek what is outside of them to make them feel better: OOOOH look at this shiny morsel over here, what about this new sexy person over there, let me have some more of that scrummy thing again and again and again. This is when pleasure-seeking becomes an unhealthy sticking plaster for the I-am-not-enough wound. When we choose tools which bring us deeper into relationship with ourselves, be it meditation, Reiki, therapy, yoga, recovery groups, or spending time with elders, it becomes easier to believe that seeking pleasurable highs is not what will keep us alive. I heard author Anna Sansom say recently that pleasure need not be a 'peak experience'. I love that. In other words, pleasure needn't be the seeking of a high, but can be savoured in everyday stuff. How about the flowers seen on your route to work or a simple, nourishing meal you cook for yourself?

A lot needs to happen to help an addict stay off their drug of choice, be it heroin or shopping. This is outside the scope of this book. I have provided signposting to recovery tools at the back of the book. However, I know that had I not become aware of my belief that I was not enough, and learned to trust that what I thought I needed in external pleasure-seeking could be found in my relationship with myself, I would probably still be using. I would probably still be what is known in some Buddhist lineages as a 'hungry ghost'. A person who is barely connected with their physical body with a bottomless gaping hole for a belly that they strive to fill via addictive tendencies. The ghost needs to get more, do more and be more to satiate the profound hunger of believing they are not enough, a hunger that instead needs to be fed with radical self-care.

There was not enough pleasure from all the drugs or pleasure of validation from all the sex that would have made me feel enough, whole. I hate the ickiness of the cliché I am about to write, but, deep breath, here goes:

staying off cocaine (amongst other things) helped me to discover that I already had everything I needed. I could, in fact, cope without it.

It is your relationship with yourself that will reveal your wholeness.

Rising

What conditioning have you soaked up concerning the role of women in sex?

Describe a woman who is too much when it comes to sex. Describe a woman who is not enough.

What impact has this had on your enjoyment of sex? Perhaps there have been positive and negative effects ...

Does pleasure feel like something you can safely receive?

What kind of touch feels good on your body? If you are unsure, how might you find out?

Does it feel OK to listen to what shame may have to tell you?

How do you feel about asking for what you want? Maybe it is easier to ask for some things and not others: more milk for your tea, another biscuit or dessert, time away from your children, a foot massage, a pay increase, oral sex?

Being honest with yourself, are there pleasurable activities you engage in that actually cause you harm?

How do you feel about not engaging in this activity?

Remember to look at the recovery resources if you think you may be dealing with addiction.

Some women want to have sex so they can have a baby. Others could not think of anything worse than getting pregnant. Do you want to be a mum?

Reclaim your pleasure.

I dare you.

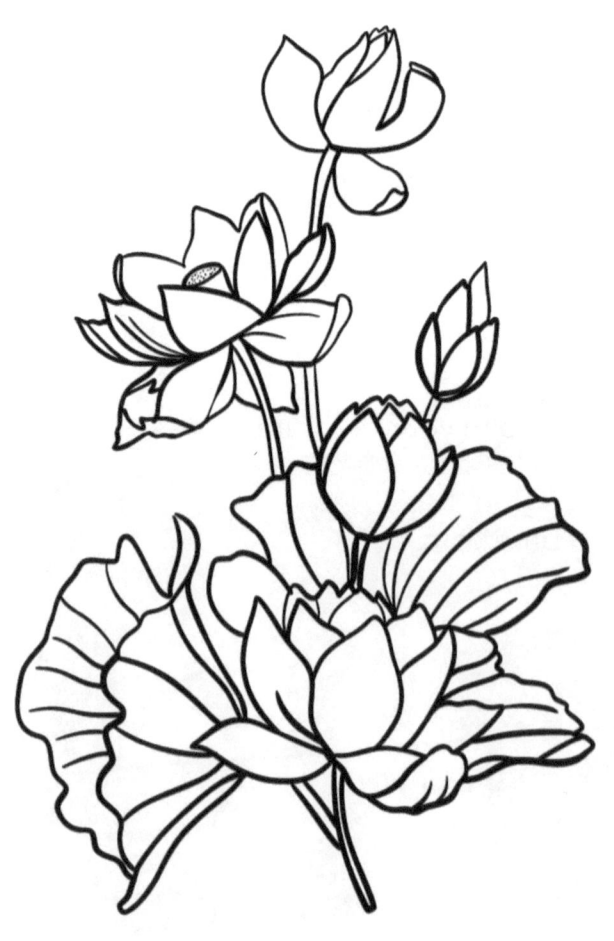

CHAPTER TWELVE

To Mum or Not To Mum. That is the Question...

Rest

Before a foray into the mum zone, take a chill pill and lean into this chapter's rest practice on youreenoughyoga.com.

Recovery

The rain was pelting onto the metal roof of Leeds train station, huge sheets of water raining down like the special effects in a disaster film. I was featuring in my own private disaster flick, closeted away in the station toilets where the air hung heavy and even the women's toilet stank of stale piss. I sat on the toilet, bent almost double and hands quivering as I struggled to unwrap the little test kit. My breath was shallow, ragged. This was long before I had learned to calm myself with the magical tools of slow breath and meditation. This was the first pregnancy test out of the three I had bought. Whatever the result was, I needed to be sure. The man I should not have been fucking didn't know that I was crouched over this smelly loo in Leeds station. He did not know that I thought I might be pregnant. He was not going to know either. I was on the pill, so it was unlikely that one of his swimmers had made it through, but nevertheless, I was shit scared that I was pregnant and it would 100% be his. If the result was positive, I wouldn't be keeping it. He would never know about the three tests and the tears in my eyes, the sweat on my back and my pounding heart, my ragged breath and racing mind. The liquid penetrated the test paper in the swab.

As far back as I can remember, I never wanted to be a mum. It is as simple as that. As simple as Henry Hill in the film *Goodfellas* stating,

'As far back as I can remember, I always wanted to be a gangster.'

I love how Goodfellas opens with teenage Henry being propelled into the air by an explosion he had just set for the New York mob. I can't ever see myself literally blowing stuff up but it's safe to say that I feel as strongly about my choice to be childfree as Henry felt about impressing his boss. If I daydream a film about what it means to be a woman, it would be a dystopia with a vigilante guerrilla woman leaping into the air after setting an explosion at a human hatchery similar to those in Aldous Huxley's *Brave*

New World, set against a voiceover drily stating: *as far back as I can remember, I always wanted to be childless.*

As a woman who has elected to be childless, it seems like society concludes that women like me who choose to stay out of Mumville must be either ill or unable to have kids or both. Or worse, we must be total bitches. Surely it is not a lot to ask for the collective to get its head around the simple fact that there are women who just do not want to have children. End of. The choice to mum or not to mum is a patriarchal minefield of too much and not enough. An ex-partner declared during the death spasms of our relationship:

'You are not a REAL woman, you don't even want to have children.'

Ouch. No surprises as to why we were breaking up. For sure, his words were a projection of his disappointment about what he thought was his right – to impregnate me – coupled with his confusion that it was not simply a given that I wanted to be a mum. He had never considered before that I may not want my womb to be a spawning station waiting to be inhabited just because society tells me that it should be. For me, my body is not a place that I want to be inhabited or infiltrated by anything that I do not 100% want to be there, including semen, a foetus, and, thanks to our current zeitgeist, experimental gene therapy jabs. It's such an old-school feminist trope, but here goes: women have the right to say what happens with our bodies. If a woman wants to have a baby, brilliant. There are enough women who do want to get knocked up that the human race has no danger of dying out. But who knows, the dinosaurs probably thought they would be around forever too? Mother Earth will decide when our time is up.

This is Not Nice and Not Pretty

I'm about to say something that I think will make me rather unpopular, I feel vulnerable even writing it and feel the clamour of a mob with pitchforks aloft, all baying for my blood. *Remember our witches,* I say to myself. Ok, just need to exhale. Here it is: I find the idea of pregnancy utterly revolting, and I just do not find the idea of motherhood to be an attractive one. I used to spend a long time judging myself, worrying I was a horrible freak for having this opinion. I used to try to make myself and my opinion more palatable. Have you ever done that, given a watered-down, nice version of what you really think and feel about something in order to make yourself seem less fired up and more agreeable? I would water it down by saying that one day I might adopt a child. This smoke-screen response would kill two birds with one stone: A) it left open the possibility that I might be a mum one day, and B) it bought me kudos for doing something humanitarian while covering up what I believed was my shameful truth. I knew I would never be having children. The good news is that I am not a horrible freak for feeling this way, and it does not make me less of a woman. It just means my opinion is a tad unorthodox but I am not wrong for having it. It is not even because I don't like kiddos. I used to be a one-to-one teacher, so I definitely do have a soft spot for the younglings. I was queen of getting teary-eyed over pupils having those lightbulb moments when they suddenly understood what on Earth Shakespeare was trying to say or that it was OK to write that Phillip Larkin's poetry was the most depressing thing they'd ever seen. Those were precious moments in English class when teenagers understood that they were allowed to have their own views about the stuff they were made to read. Being a teacher does not mean that I would ever want to have my own offspring, though. Does my choice to be childless mean I am not enough, not a proper woman? Does it mean I am too much, too unpalatable for patriarchal society? What do you think? Tell the truth.

Needless to say that I fully support my friends who want to be pregnant or are already parents. Motherhood seems to suit my friends. I just know it is not for me. I find myself slipping into norms when women tell me they are pregnant. 'Congratulations!' The word falls out of my mouth unconsciously. Is each woman I have congratulated genuinely happy to be pregnant? I wonder what would happen if I could rewind time and ask if they are happy about it. It feels edgy just thinking about doing that. What would happen? A slap in the face? Maybe. Many would say, 'Yes, of course I'm happy.' Some would say, 'No, I'm not happy. I want to get rid of it.' It would be pretty boundaryless of me to ask that of somebody I did not really know, so I will probably give it a miss. I like to think that I could hold space for a friend to tell me if she wasn't sure motherhood was for her. For me, the choice to have an abortion epitomises what it is to be a courageous woman in a world which presumes you would be happy to have a baby whenever. Then again, I have friends who openly say they were not ready to have their baby, but they also can't say what 'ready' really looks like, so maybe they were ready and they simply did not realise. It's just different strokes for different folks. I don't believe there is anything about choosing to mum or not to mum that makes a woman too much or not enough.

Are you wondering why I do not want to be a mum? *What was your childhood like? What is your relationship with your mum like?* These are the classic unsolicited questions I have been asked both by friends and randoms when I have revealed confidently that motherhood is not for me. Would people pry unsolicited into the psychology of a man who wanted to be childfree? Just a thought. A friend told me that it was a shame that I did not want to be a mum, and perhaps I should look into this with my therapist to make sure I don't miss out on a wonderful experience. I disagree that motherhood would be a wonderful experience, from what I have observed, motherhood looks profoundly stressful, unfair, and has the potential for a woman to judge herself as being not enough or too much cranked up to the max. As it happened, the subject does get broached when I have therapy; nothing that I have discovered has changed my mind. If anything, it has made my choice more resolute. This friend was desperate to be a mum, and more and more, she would act out her confusion and annoyance toward me that I simply did not want the same thing she wanted. We have parted company.

It Starts at Conception

From what I can gather, the curse of too much and not enough infiltrates a mum's life before a child is even born! *Are you taking enough supplements? Have you had too much to drink? Have you read insert-name-of-parenting-book? Home birth or hospital, no drugs or all the drugs? (Whatever you choose, there will be somebody who implies that your choice is wrong.) Are you and baby's dad getting married now? Are you cutting out X and eating more of X? Vaginal birth or elective caesarean? You're getting your children vaccinated, right?* Get ready to justify and defend your choice. Or not. Of course, nobody has to defend or justify any of their choices about birth or motherhood ever, but society and the medical establishment expect us to. I like to think that the imaginary pregnant Sarah would tell the pregnancy inquisition to Fuck Right Off (more politely, if the circumstances required it!), but maybe I would feel the societal pressure to give all the normative right answers too. Probably.

When the long-awaited birth is over, the lifelong labour to raise a child begins. There are the myriad decisions to make about the welfare of the tiny creature, and the direction its life needs to take according to the hopes and dreams of its parents. These hopes and dreams may not be the same hopes and dreams of the tiny human who will be influenced from the moment it is born as to how it must behave to be an acceptable citizen, strive to be good enough and not cause too much trouble. Fuck that. I would hate to be burdened with the creeping anxiety that somehow I would inadvertently damage the child, a cross word on a stressed-out day triggering psychological harm to the little one. Children's brains are so vulnerable because they are so attuned to the emotional state of the parents, like little sponges who soak up the fallout of everyday stressors. There is the risk of childhood trauma, a subject again too huge for the scope of this book and best explained by experts like Dr Gabor Matē. When a parent inadvertently or purposefully rejects, abandons, or shames the child as a result of the parent's own unexplored trauma, the impact on the child is deeply detrimental to their development. Honestly, being a mum looks so hard and I am not ashamed to admit that it scares me. The freedom of being childless is something I am unwilling to give up. I recall something validating that my therapist said,

'Every woman needs a lifetime that is purely just for them.'

Perhaps in my soul's next life, I will be first in the motherhood queue! But right now, I am reminded of the visceral relief of the three negative tests I took in the piss-stinking toilet.

It must be the Woman, Right?

Patriarchy is geared to give men an easier time than women. Fact. This pattern continues when the issue of motherhood is brooded upon. The inequality begins with the biological fact that the bloke will not be impregnated but is the impregnator, which seems to win him much respect for the simple biology of ejaculating inside a vagina. I've seen men get a slap on the back and a 'nice one, mate' when they announce that success of their ejaculation inside a woman and she has become pregnant. For men, ejaculating is not particularly difficult, but the successful impregnation apparently proves his functional Masculinity and his worth as a male. When a man is infertile, he is said to be 'firing blanks', implying that his sperm is empty, in effect, not manly sperm. This idiom shames men. This shaming demonstrates the backward nature of patriarchy's subtle attack on men as well as women. Under patriarchy, ineffectual sperm = ineffectual man, says society. However, when the ammo has hit the target of achieving the pregnancy, it is full steam ahead for the pressure and inconvenience that women face. The bloke goes down the pub, but the woman looks forward to nine months (if the baby is punctual, friends tell me it is nearer nine and a half months) of hormone rollercoaster accompanied by a glut of physical, emotional, and mental symptoms while society still expects her to be a fully functioning partner/unpaid housekeeper/lover/career queen/birth planner all while making a watertight plan to get back into her pre-baby jeans after the birth.

In my humble, non-expert, non-mum opinion, I think women need to have three years of fully paid leave to get their minds and bodies recovered from birth, to take some space to enjoy being a parent. Men need proper paternity leave too, so they can support their partner with all the extra life admin that comes with being a parent. Obviously, this applies to same-sex couples too. Proper time off for all new parents, please! From what I have observed from my friends, it seems that fathers are not spending as much time with their new offspring as the mothers, which leaves them ignorant of what really goes on in a day in the life of a new mum. Fathers need to see what is happening so they can offer greater levels of empathy and support. On the flipside, if mum wants to trot back into work a couple of weeks after giving birth, then she should crack on with no judgement from society about her choice to swerve the domestic chores of new motherhood.

Ouch

I am reliably informed by friends that staying with your baby all the time is very, very boring. In perfect synchronicity, while I was sat typing this piece in a café, a couple of women were chatting about motherhood and how surprised they are that one of their mates is resolute in her choice not to have children after one of their other friends was terribly injured giving birth in hospital. They were discussing that her inner genitalia 'tore and completely collapsed.' Surely you would look at your kid and be like, 'Thanks.'

People who raise children astound me with their patience, resilience, and joy they seem to feel from parenting. It is honestly heart-warming and awesome, so those people who genuinely want to get all babied up should go right ahead, as long as they are fully capable of looking after their children with no hint of physical or emotional neglect. In my previous job as a teacher for young people with severe behaviour and emotional issues, I saw the real-life effects of childhood abuse and trauma. The signs and symptoms of abuse are endless: cigarette burns on skin, bruising, autoimmune conditions, self-harm, aggression toward other children, cruelty to animals, speech impediments, inability to trust or too much trust, cognitive difficulties, C-PTSD, ADHD, inappropriately sexualised behaviour, zero self-esteem, agoraphobia, physical ticks, Tourette's syndrome, special educational needs, digestion problems, lice, etc. There are people who should not be parents because they cannot properly look after their children. The damage inflicted on the child will be lifelong if no intervention is made to heal the effects of abuse with genuine care and nurture. All of this being said, for those women who do choose to be mums and are offering their kids the kind of 'entry-level mothering' described by Julia on the hilarious comedy *Motherland*, my wish is that these women break free from the societal expectations of perfection that are loaded onto them from the moment they conceive. Children just need proper care, love, and attention, they do not need their mums to be superheroes. For us gals who are avoiding motherhood like the plague, let's keep remembering that we are more than enough without a couple of kids in tow.

Rising

Have you ever felt pressured to have a baby? If so, where or whom did the pressure come from?

Has the experience of feeling like you are too much or not enough influenced your choice to have/not to have children?

What do you think about women who choose to be childfree? Let the judgements out on to your page – they are only societal conditioning, after all!

What do you think of women who choose to have children? Again, allow the judgements to flow out ...

Should women be paid for the work of motherhood?

If you are a mum, explore your experience of giving birth. Perhaps you want to write, draw, or collage on this question.

If you are planning to have children, what are your fears about motherhood? What you are most looking forward to?

What did you need to hear from your caregivers that you never heard?

Wow, this chapter has felt like A LOT. Fancy some retail therapy?

It is OK to stop to breathe.

You have done enough.

You are doing enough.

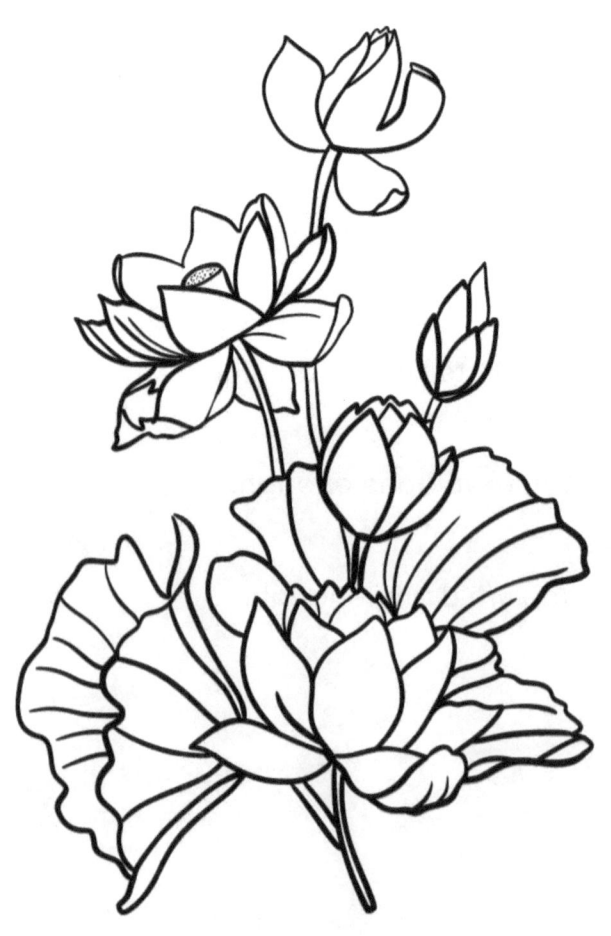

CHAPTER THIRTEEN

Enoughness for Sale

Rest

This chapter has a slightly different resting practice. Sit comfortably and meditate on some warm, loving, enoughness feelings over on the Enough! area of my website.

Recovery

Patriarchy's curse influences us to buy shit that we don't need to help us feel we are enough. We buy the obligatory smartphone because everybody has one and because technology moves so fucking fast that you need one to keep up with all the scanning of QR codes, counting our steps on the fitness app, and posting photos of picture-perfect offspring or vegan brunches to Instagram for a habitual dopamine hit. I really try to avoid doing those things! Both capitalism and one-upmanship have conditioned people to keep up with the metaphorical Joneses. It does not take a genius to look at the phrase 'one-upmanship' to see the patriarchal influence behind it, its energy driven by 'get more, get better, prove oneself or get crushed beneath the man who has the competitive edge'. That's my read on it, anyway. Here is what a dictionary has to say: 'One-upmanship is defined as the practice of always trying to be better than or gain superiority over others.'

'An example of one-upmanship is when you wait to announce your wife is pregnant until the dinner at which your brother announces he is engaged, just to take the attention off of your brother.' https://www.yourdictionary.com/one-upmanship

This is such a brilliantly unsurprising example of patriarchal one-upmanship! There's the familiar patriarchal flavour of superiority, of unrelentingly trying to be better than the next person, or if the example is anything to go by, the next man. Men are at the centre of this example while the invisible fiancé (who I am guessing is female because of the heteronormative tone of the example) and the pregnant wife are women who are being shown off – one as an item of property by one brother, and the other as the vessel for the other brother's developing child. The brother with the pregnant wife is the winner in the yukky example because he has a wife AND she is pregnant. He and his mate have proved their virility and fertility, and he has ticked more boxes than his brother on the hypothetical successful demonstration of manliness chart Own woman: check! Impregnate her: check! Being one step ahead or owning the preferred, coveted item and status is the conditioned toxic masculine way of supposedly winning at life. This behaviour has crept into the majority of Western societal living, whether you are a man with a pregnant wife to show off, a teen with the latest iPhone to drool over, a wellness fiend with membership at the best wellness centre or an aspiring beauty blogger with the expensive lip gloss. Pretty much everybody wants the newest, biggest, best, more expensive something and we have to get it fast. If we can't afford a designer bag/coat/lip gloss that's OK – just get a really cheap version, right? Somehow people developed an aversion to OK, to possessions that are simply good enough or that do not resemble the biggest, best, expensive brands. At the time of writing this chapter, it is Black Friday weekend which will be followed by Cyber Monday. I swear if I receive one more email enticing me into last-minute Black Friday sales, I will end up screaming into a pillow. I think it is time to unsubscribe from thirsty brands who bombard me with email marketing day after day. Yuk. It can be a struggle to remember that above the clamouring noise of the online marketplace, we probably do not even want what they are selling, be it sleek, overpriced yoga gear or shiny techy gadgets.

Patriarchy and capitalism have successfully tempted people to associate our intrinsic worth with the items we own.

The Human Cost of Shop-Bought Enoughness

It seems as if the supposed life hack is to make sure you get the best of everything, or the most of everything, or both, regardless of the costs.

Forget about the children who mine the cobalt for the inner mechanics of the latest smartphone.[1]

Forget about Amazon's exploitative labour practices of warehouse workers where the items we need in a hurry are stored.[2]

Forget about the outsourced sweatshop labour needed to make expensive brand yoga clothes in factories which pressure workers to refrain from taking breaks to meet the demand for clothing by Western buyers.[3]

Forget about the women factory workers in Bangladesh who are emotionally and physically abused by supervisors; 'women at the bottom of supply chains bear the brunt of fashion's unrelenting push to be fast and cheap …' says Anna Bryher from Labour Behind the Label, quoted in *The Guardian's* article exposing yoga clothing brand Lululemon.[4]

Forget the people crushed in the Bangladesh Rana Plaza disaster in 2013, making our cheap, unethical fad fashion.[5]

Do you find it easy to forget about the people who suffer to make the things that we want?

Let's take a breather here. I've just reeled off a lot of information about where stuff comes from, and I notice writing this, I am feeling ashamed of being too much, of saying too much about things that are unpleasant, hard to digest. That is my conditioning at play. But I am not too much. I care and want to tell people so that we can make choices that do not fuck people over, particularly people who are already economically underprivileged thanks to patriarchy's darlings: racism, misogyny, and control.

Patriarchy taught us one-upmanship, and when people act on it, the underprivileged people suffer. In our insatiable quest to look the part or have the best stuff, to get it quickly so we can wear and use these things to show that we are enough, that we ourselves are valuable, unseen people suffer and die. I am not rich, but I do sometimes have money to spare on clothes, and I used to be a regular Primark shopper. I enjoyed feeling like was getting some good deals on pretty dresses, snazzy make-up, and basics that didn't cost the Earth – except they do. They cost people and nature. It's hard because I think my brain enjoyed the dopamine hit of walking out of Primark each week with a new outfit, my little reward for working hard, to help me remember that I looked anything from nice to sexy to sporty to smart, a doll with my own wardrobe bursting with different looks. I am pretty sure that I swapped cocaine for shopping in my late twenties, but I'm happy to say that my dopamine-driven spending has ceased.

Spirituality for Sale

The wellness industry, which comprises the monetisation of spirituality and health, is an attractive place for Westerners who have money to spend. A quick internet search reveals that the US and UK wellness market is estimated to be worth around sixty billion dollars. Spiritual systems from around the world and health trends are both romanticised and reduced to glittery yoga mats; sacred symbols and script misappropriated and printed onto yoga vests; dream catchers made in China sold in new age gift shops; pricey crystal pendants marketed on the strong suggestion they CAN absolutely heal trauma. (I would really love to believe this about crystals but perhaps a person could seek out therapy too, to cover all bases!) If you have ever been to a yoga studio which has a shop, you may have looked at the pretty mala beads on sale which people may or may not be purchasing for their traditional meditational use, the leggings which cost at least £50 (with no visible guarantee they have not been made by using sweatshop labour), and the diffusers puffing out deliciously spicy, aspirational essential oil aromas while customers sign in for class. There is nothing wrong with buying yourself treats, and I think it is every woman's right to adorn herself with beautiful objects. There is something ancient, Feminine, and ritualistic about wearing jewellery, be it expensive or not. What is interesting to me, though, is the phenomenon that wafts around the wellness world which may be the motivating or more sinister, coercive force behind spending on the stuff at the wellness fair or yoga studio's lifestyle store ...

I used to buy A LOT of this stuff: Buddha and Ganesh ornaments (any kind of Buddha: fat ones, laughing ones, reclining ones or Siddhartha sitting in meditation), essential oils (because they must have healing properties, right? The enormous multi-level marketing companies that sell them surely would not lie to make millions in profit?), vitamins and supplements so I could achieve optimum health (I swung from the striving of anorexia to striving to be as well as possible!), a special 'life-saving' gadget which was basically just a shiny foil sticker for my smart phone to ward off high levels of electromagnet frequency (yeah, I could have just used my phone less) – the list goes on. Any of this sounding familiar?

For a long while, I believed the hype that owning these kinds of trinkets would reinforce the identity that I was constructing for myself: spiritual seeker with sexy, earthy glam. However, the deeper into relationship with myself that my spiritual practices took me, I realised that I did not need to show off my spiritual nature to the world. It sounds so obvious to say it now, but nobody needs special clothes or a pricey mat to practice yoga. These things become part of an identikit image peddled to us by the wellness industry to make us buy their stuff. Yep, they play on our insecurities that we may not be enough and hey presto, their gear can help us believe that we are enough. Remember those hungry ghosts? Except it does not work because the outside stuff does not repair the inner wound of believing oneself not to be good enough. The wound repairing happens on the inside, and more than likely in private with a patient therapist or the care of a healer. I absolutely believe that clothes can help show who we are and can lend a whole truckload of creative self-expression into our daily lives. I simply swoon when Tan France on *Queer Eye* huge-heartedly helps a person pick a new wardrobe to suit the glorious person underneath the clothes. Yet our clothes, accessories, and gadgets do not need to be the costume we put on to prove our enoughness to the outside world.

Rising

What items of clothing do you use to prove that you are good enough, confident, clever, sexy, wealthy, spiritual, climate conscious, Feminist, etc? Could you continue to be and feel these things if you lost those items from your wardrobe?

Are there items you spend money on that you think you need but that you do not really get happiness from?

Is there something you are trying to prove when you spend money on material goods?

Do you shop to cheer yourself up?

When was the first time you remember wanting something (a product) to make yourself feel better?

Are there times when you believe your enoughness or self-worth is connected to the money you spend or the products you buy?

Do you spend money because you feel you are worth it?

Do you spend money to make you believe you are worth it?

It is so tempting to try to buy our enoughness or go looking for it, credit card in hand. I have totally done that. If you do that too, don't beat yourself up.

Has your search for enoughness led you toward any unpleasant folk? Let's explore the heady blend of chemistry concocted when 'I'm not good enough' meets toxic people.

All of these whispers humming around my brain and body. I read it all in black and white, categorising the things he did. Abusive behaviours. All remembered by my pain. I am told that the past cannot hurt me …

Not true.

But no more, no way. I am my own person, not your prey.

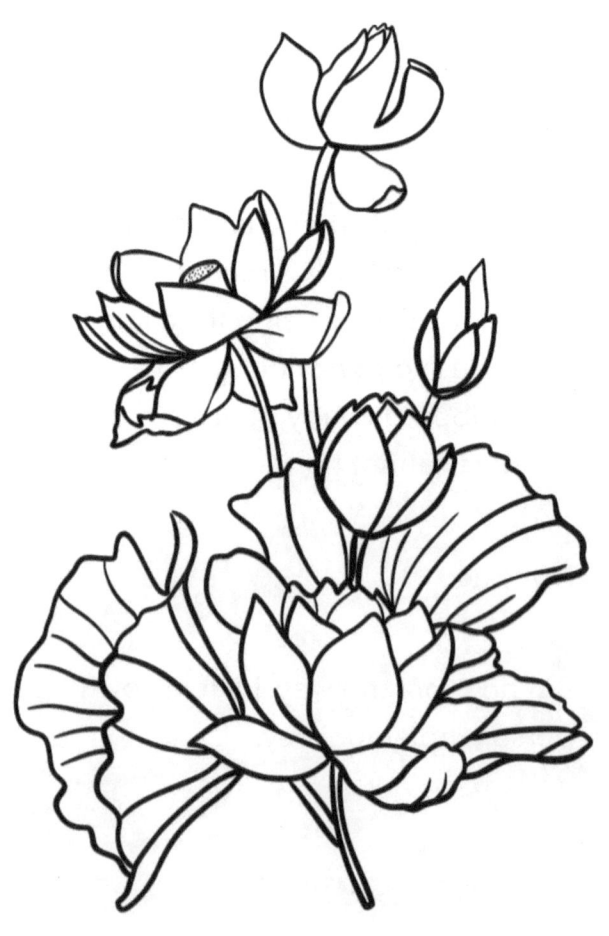

CHAPTER FOURTEEN

It Is Not All in Your Head

Rest

This week, you'll connect your body to the Earth in your Yoga Nidrā practice.

Recovery

Sometimes it seems that the entire structure of Western society plays into propagating patriarchy's curse of too much and not enough. When we return home from education or work, switch off our techy devices, unplug from the news and turn toward our closest relationships, we are looking for safe havens. We need relationships with others and ourselves that allow us to feel enough, safe, heard, respected, and nourished. Unfortunately, many women have experienced relationship patterns which are the opposite of these basic relational requirements and instead endured the perpetration of abusive behaviours against us. I call these behaviours toxic because abusive relationships are bad for our health. Of course, anybody is vulnerable to relational abuse and this is terribly sad. However, reports show that in England and Wales, more than 90% of those being abused are women. A large proportion of these women report that the first instance of domestic abuse happened while they were pregnant.[1] Being on the receiving end of behaviour patterns such as gaslighting, manipulation, lying, invalidation, verbal abuse, shaming, coercive control, withholding affection, defamation, financial abuse, undermining, triangulation, silent treatment, and physical violence is painful and poisonous to our necessary belief that we are enough.

Abusers Steal Our Sense of Enoughness

Abuse can be physical, emotional, or psychological and for some survivors, their perpetrator serves up a mix of all three. Only recently, society came to terms with the fact that it is wrong to beat your spouse, and that sex without consent in a relationship is most definitely rape (I face-plant my head into my hand in disbelief that this even needs explaining). The Domestic Abuse Bill, which includes the outlawing of coercive control, only came into effect in 2020. The charity Women's Aid states that domestic abuse is a gendered crime because this type of abuse disproportionately affects women. We are on the receiving end of abuse simply because we are women.

Emotional and psychological abuse against women is a scourge that leaves survivors feeling confused, frightened, demeaned, self-doubting, violated, boundaryless, hopeless and helpless while both instilling and reinforcing fear in the survivor that they are not enough, their emotions are too much, their emotions and needs do not matter, safety is not their right, they cannot get anything right and do not deserve love and respect. Survivors may eventually leave an abusive relationship (which is so damn hard to do) only to unconsciously find themselves in other relationships in which abuse against them is repeated. It is known that abuse survivors can cycle back into relationships which harm them due to the familiarity that hurt and relational chaos can evoke. Getting sucked into harmful relationships is an unconscious process, and I will say it LOUDER for anybody who is unsure, abuse survivors do not manifest nor intentionally seek out more abuse.

The trauma caused by abuse has a lasting impact, and some survivors (like myself) may have been unconsciously snared by or stayed with people who intend to harm them because of the familiar energetic pattern of harm which is held in the body. Somebody told me once that intense 'chemistry' and strong attraction that almost feels compulsive, like an addiction, between people is, in fact, past trauma being triggered. Sure, not all strong attraction is a red flag for potential toxicity in a relationship, but if this attraction is paired with love-bombing (a person's constant need to hook your attention, acted out by hundreds of texts, extravagant gifts and holidays early in a relationship) from the object of your desire or an exciting new friend, take a breath and take note. We only need to look at the fallout of serial abuser 'Simon Leviev' in the documentary *The Tinder Swindler* to see the lengths that abusers will go to in order to hook their prey. If someone is whisking you off to different countries for date number one, see the red flag! Love-bombing is a type of grooming in emotional abuse to trick victims into believing that the abuser is a good person who will always treat them well. Sadly, as time passes, love-bombing gives way to behaviour patterns such as undermining, criticising, manipulation, gaslighting, and discarding, all key features in the playbook of narcissistic abuse.

Narcissistic abuse and narcissistic personality styles are so common; in fact, they are both normalised and admired in Western society. Patriarchy favours people who fight their way into positions of power in both blatant cut-throat fashion and by corrupt, underhand scheming. The system lauds power, and power is what feeds narcissistic personality styles. Just look at government and politics, full of people fighting to get into power, and when they get some power, it is not enough (because narcissists can never be satiated), so they salivate for more power and carry out in-fighting and corruption within their own political parties. Check out the relationships demonstrated in Britain's Conservative party in 2021: Boris Johnson versus Dominic Cummings, Cummings versus Matt Hancock, Hancock cheating on his wife by shagging his younger intern.

Power Hungry

Now consider the vile behaviour of convicted creeps like Jeff Epstein, Harvey Weinstein, and Bernie Madoff. All people desperate to maintain power to inflate and protect their egos via abusing others and attempting to rob people of their power. To be clear, I am not diagnosing any of the named persons as narcissists because being narcissistic is not itself a diagnosis. It is a description. Plus, I am not a psychologist, so I can't be diagnosing anything! Despite my lack of medical expertise, I am not afraid to use these terms, though, and I don't care if I am labelled judgemental for doing so. Naming narcissistic abuse gave me a blueprint for recognising the behaviour perpetrated against me, for what it actually was: abuse. Survivors need to name what has happened to us so that we can heal. HUGE CAVEAT: If you have a narcissist in your life, do not call out the narcissist to the narcissist! That's what psychologists say definitely not to do! You might be itching to tell them you have them figured out and their game is up, but it only goes one way for the truth-teller and that is badly. There are tons of resources online to help cope with, understand, and extricate from narcissistic abuse, so you may like to peruse these to help you take care of yourself. Back to terminology. 'Narcissistic' and 'narcissism' are descriptions of behaviour patterns which are self-serving, scheming, manipulative, and invalidating of others. I am pointing to their patterns of accumulating power and control to reinforce their egos while harming others. Narcissism is dangerous and made all the more sinister because it is so commonplace. I can't speak on behalf of Epstein and Weinstein's victims/survivors, but seeing these perpetrators get away with it for so long because they were lauded by glitzy society must have been beyond tough and the ultimate form of tribal gaslighting.

We have been taught to admire the driven go-getters who always make it to the top. Not all successful, rich go-getters are narcissistic but many narcistic individuals have indeed become rich and powerful at the expense of emotionally abusing people on their way to the top, particularly those with grandiose narcissism traits (think *Wolf of Wall Street*) and those with malignant narcissism traits (think Epstein). What gets left in the wake of this abuse are swathes of people struggling to recover from the long-term effects of psychological and physical harm; confidence knocked, nervous system destabilised, slowly recovering their belief in themselves and their worth.

Narcissism has become a buzzword in recent years. I like to think that this is because people are getting wise to the behaviours displayed by the various types of narcissists, be they grandiose, malignant or covert in their personality style. Yep, there are different styles of narcissists and for deeper insight and expertise around these styles, please refer to the work of clinical psychologist and narcissism specialist Dr Ramani Durvasula. Dr Ramani's work has been a godsend in my own understanding of and recovery from narcissistic abuse. More and more survivors of narcissistic abuse are courageously coming forward to help raise awareness of these insidious abuse patterns that can leave survivors trapped for years in toxic relationships, whether this be with a narcissist family member, partner, friend, boss, spiritual leader, coach or therapist. Being emotionally abused by a narcissist is a breeding ground for instilling not-enoughness into the victim. Forcing a person to question their worth is the narcissist's prize for protecting and fluffing up their own ego. *Wait, you may say, don't narcissists already have massive egos without any extra fluff?* Actually, no, they act like they have strong egos but the narcissist is fragile and cannot handle any kind of constructive criticism or feedback, and so to avoid this kryptonite at all costs, they cruelly fling vindictive, abusive behaviour at their victims to make them believe they are not enough. Narcissists feed like vampires by invalidating their victims. I have crossed paths with a few narcissists in my time, and it has not been pretty. What they had in common was their desperately fragile egos that they strived to protect by devaluing those around them, and in my intimate relations with a narcissist, it was me they zeroed in on to invalidate.

Rescuing Leaves Us Vulnerable to Vampires

Nobody wants to be with people who abuse them and make them feel like a piece of shit, but these patterns die hard, particularly if you recognise yourself as a 'rescuer'. I used to be a rescuer. I believed that if I could just show enough love, patience, acceptance, and positivity to my former narcissistic/emotional abusers, then I would be able to rescue these people who treated me badly, rescuing them from themselves and their unacceptable behaviour. A life in which the leopard (the abuser) changes their spots. People who abuse in a narcissistic behaviour style do not change, but it can take years for survivors to let this undesirable fact drop into place, and even longer to summon their courage to leave the relationship. Truthfully though, not all abuse survivors can completely extricate themselves from the relationship with their narcissistic abuser particularly if there are matters of financial security and/or co-parenting. I'm glad to say there are many online resources to help a person develop boundaries to cope with the narcissist if they are unable to totally end the relationship. Boundaries or out and out leaving will help an abuse survivor's energy tank start to refill. It is true, I felt fuller, more grounded each time I moved my energy away from these unhealthy relationships.

I am damn sure that patriarchal society taught me to be a rescuer and primed me to accept toxic behaviour; in other words, to be the perfect partner/friend who set such a good example by being bloody lovely all the time and co-dependently doing so much for everyone, including the abusive person, that they would realise how much they needed me and start being nice to me. Remember what I said about Brownies a few chapters ago? 'I promise to lend a hand and put other people before myself.' Yikes.

I would make excuses for my ex-partners and ex-friends who treated me like crap. *Oh, I know he/she does not mean it. It is just their suppressed childhood anger coming out. They had such a hard childhood and that's why they say those things. He is right, I have been too emotional lately and I know it makes him uncomfortable. It's just words and words can't hurt me. Don't be too hard on her, she is going through a rough time. If I can just find a new tactic to ask him to talk about his feelings, then it will get better. I know it will get better. He promised he won't do it again. I need to believe in him more so he can change. It's probably just my perception upsetting me, I shouldn't have got upset. Must be more positive so I can inspire him. Got to raise my vibration so there is no negativity between us. I know it sounded like a threat but their bark is worse than their bite. He doesn't like red lipstick, I will only wear it when I'm out with my friends.* No matter what I told myself or the people who tried to help me see sense that my rationalising and excuses were enabling my abusers, underneath all the justifications was a heavy, sludgy feeling of stagnating fear coupled with my belief that I deserved what was happening. I thought I was not enough to deserve better. The fear was real, it was not all in my head – so real that being in toxic relationships undermined my health and vitality by conjuring panic attacks, tension headaches, and digestion trouble.

Shut Your Mouth

Perfection rears its destructive head again. I tried to prove that being the perfect partner/friend/colleague would somehow melt away the abusive behaviour, that being a shiny example of a forgiving, patient, sweet-natured woman would denature the toxicity that abusers sent my way. I believe that expectations placed upon women by society prime us to tolerate unacceptable or abusive behaviour from those we are in relationship with. History has taught us to keep silent, literally forcing our mouths closed with the punishment of a scold's bridle if a woman dared to say a bad word about her husband, another woman, or an authority figure, or simply spoke in a way that a judge deemed out of turn. Put up and shut up. If you are unsure what a scold's bridle is, it is a metal clamp designed to be worn on the face to hold the tongue in place to stop the 'scold' (the woman) from speaking. This misplaced tolerance for abuse perhaps increases if you happen to come from a religious or spiritual background. Why? Because Jesus teaches us to love our neighbours, turn the other cheek (literally to get another slap), have patience, forgive and pray for our enemies. There is nothing wrong with kindness, of course, or forgiveness when actioned by the forgiver as an autonomous act to free themselves from resentment. Yet Bible stories, religious tropes and new age spirituality can keep an abuse cycle running while women pray for the person who beats and/or gaslights them, offering their perpetrator the spiritual gift of unconditional love.

I have learned that love has no room for abuse, love is not supposed to hurt and a healthy relationship will not have me feeling strung out or uncomfortable.

I have never considered myself religious, thanks to my smart move to quit Sunday school as a seven-year-old, so I have not been indoctrinated to tolerate abuse against me on religious grounds. But my mingling in the personal development and spiritual communities, particularly within the cults I found myself in, preached some pretty damaging views on abusive relationships.

Pardon the culty lingo while I explain this total mindfuck. The course leaders of these high-demand groups that I was part of would encourage adult survivors of childhood abuse to phone their parent or familial perpetrator and reconcile with them. The leaders would say this was, of course, not compulsory, but if the participant really wanted to move on from their difficult past, and experience results from the course, then they should accept the invitation (strong coercion) to make the call. This is manipulation, which is a key feature of cult territory. Pressure was built up by the leaders to create remarkable results, such as participants talking with and forgiving somebody who had hurt them in the past. The participant would be encouraged to acknowledge to their chosen person or potential previous abuser that they were ready to stop blaming them about hurt they perceived had been caused to them. The word 'perceived' is key here because both of my ex-cults taught that pain and hurt were mere perceptions. It does not take a long internet search to look up research that tells us trauma from abuse can manifest as physical pain and interfere with physiological systems, such as the digestive and reproductive systems, while also reinforcing chronic physical pain.[2] This makes emotional pain far more than a mere perception.

Course leaders in these cults were not required to undergo any mental health or trauma-informed training, which meant there was zero safe container for these phone calls. Crucially, nobody gets to say or imply that another person's hurt is just a perception because, for that person, their pain is real. This is gaslighting. My hurt was real but thanks to the cult, I started to believe that when my partner at that time was cold and invalidating towards me, I could not and should not feel the very real, very natural and appropriate sadness and hurt. I would hear from the leaders that I needed to take total responsibility all of the time, and I should always be the first to apologise for any conflict in my life. Near to where I live, there is a poster on the side of a school which advertises an after-school club. The poster reads:

'Always be the first to apologise.'

Needless to say, this reminds me of the cult, but it also makes me so mad thinking about the little kids apologising for shit that was not their fault! Yep, I used to apologise endlessly when my partner gaslighted and undermined me because A) I figured that it must be my fault, and B) I had to take 100% responsibility for everything and be a champion apologiser because that was what the leaders said. If I wanted a better, more effective, enjoyable life, than I needed to do what they said, right? Nope.

I have witnessed the leaders of the groups I was in convince abuse survivors that they are the problem, that bullying and control are all in their head or a skewed perception, that the survivor is the root of any dysfunction in their life rather than the trauma from abuse. And to top it all off, I've heard some Law of Attraction folks teach that survivors manifested harm done to them. This is victim-blaming central. Rewind: Nobody Manifests Their Abuse.

In these cultic groups, abusers are assuaged of any responsibility for the carnage they caused in victims' lives. Cultic groups are closed-loop systems that also assuage themselves of any responsibility for harm done by laying the maxim of 100% responsibility upon the member. One of the groups even went so far as to portray rape as not a thing, but rather a linguistic term used by women to diminish their own responsibility for how much they turn men on. If this does not make you want to scream, then I don't know what will. Go ahead, scream out loud if you want. This one is on me.

What Am I Without Them?

Abusers need their victims to believe that they are not enough. My ex-abusers (cult leaders included) tried to make me believe that my emotions did not matter, that I was not enough without their group, and would be nothing without their presence, until they got sick of me and completed the pattern of devaluing and discarding. They needed me to disconnect from the pain being caused by the frequent emotional wounding in order for the abuse cycle to continue. They needed to destroy my wants, needs, and potential so they could keep vampiring off the life support I gave them. When I left one of the cults, I was ill and disoriented. *What would I be without them?* It was the same being discarded by the narcissistic boyfriend; I was unwell, traumatised, ashamed and ruminating. Truth is, I could do what I wanted without them squeezing the joy out of my life, without their scheming, control, and mind-fuckery. It was a long while before I would consider pondering just for half a second that I was enough and I did not need them. Even under all the pain from being emotionally abused by them, I was still there, my enoughness waiting to be discovered. I was waiting for myself to come home to the sacred abode where enoughness lives. The journey home took a while, and honestly, it is still unfolding. I'll share more about this in the next chapter.

Narcissists Do Not Change

This is so much easier said than done, and maybe it's trite of me to write this, but you do not need to tolerate abuse of any kind. No amount of love, patience, positive intentions, couple's counselling, praying, affirmations, good vibes, relational tactics, second-guessing, letting them off the hook, or excuses will ever change a narcissistic person. Even therapy is unlikely to work for them long term. The impact of abuse (physical, domestic, narcissistic) is not all in your head because abusers DO intend to make other people feel like shit as a way of projecting their discomfort with their OWN personality. It's what they do. You are not being 'too sensitive'. Jesus, I have heard that little minimisey, gaslighty phrase tooooo many times. If it feels wrong and painful, then that is your reality and it may be time to reassess whether this is a relationship that is healthy for you. The impact of feeling not enough after abuse is also real, the low self-esteem, anxiety, depression, aches and pains, panic. If you recognise that there may have been a person in your life who tried to make you feel like you are not enough, seek help. Drop the excuses and rationalisations you may have made for them because they do not get to take out their OWN shit on you or other people. Cut ties and find some resources to support your recovery.

If you have believed you are not enough or too much as a result of abuse, maybe this is the beginning of the end of that belief? You don't have to go it alone in your recovery toward reclaiming your enoughness; lean into any supportive friends (friends who do not enable your abuser by rationalising or minimising their behaviour, or suggesting you do more work on you as if this will somehow magically inspire the abuser to change) and consider some therapy from a therapist well versed in the patterns of abuse cycles and its impact. What you don't want is a therapist who wants to turn it all around and suggest that real-life abuse was simply your perception; if you get a sniff of that, pick up your things and leave.

In time and in no rush, you will believe in your own potential once again or for the first time ever.

Rising

Be gentle and patient with yourself if you choose to journal or make art on these prompts ...

> *Do you have any relationships in which you feel unsettled, harmed, disrespected or invalidated? Consider your intimate, familial, friendship and workplace relationships.*
>
> *How have these relationships reinforced any belief that you are too much or not enough or both?*
>
> *When was the first time in your life that you felt emotionally harmed, and by whom?*
>
> *What might you say to a friend who confides that they are being emotionally abused? How does it feel to turn this comfort toward yourself?*
>
> *What would it be like to set boundaries in your relationships? What does saying 'No' trigger for you?*
>
> *Can you recognise any religious or spiritual teachings that may have left you vulnerable to tolerating abuse?*
>
> *What would it be like to ask for help to heal from the harm inflicted upon you, whether this is recent or childhood harm?*

You may like to try these daily recovery mantras shared with me by life coach Carol Cavalcante. How about making some art based on these words?

I am reclaiming what was taken from me.

I am bringing life back to me.

I am recharging myself.

I am able to say no.

I am able to ask questions.

I am able to set the boundaries.

Abuse is a heavy topic, yet within the careful and compassionate exploration of the heaviness, we may find the light as we heal. Take a break from reading for now, have a tea and maybe a Yoga Nidrā or some mindful movement because the next chapter is a heavy one too. I am going to tell you about my time in two cults, both of which utterly fucked my sense of enoughness. After leaving, I found ways to rebuild who I was. #sogladileft

We must treat patriarchy the way we must treat abusers.

Disengage. Set boundaries. Recover.

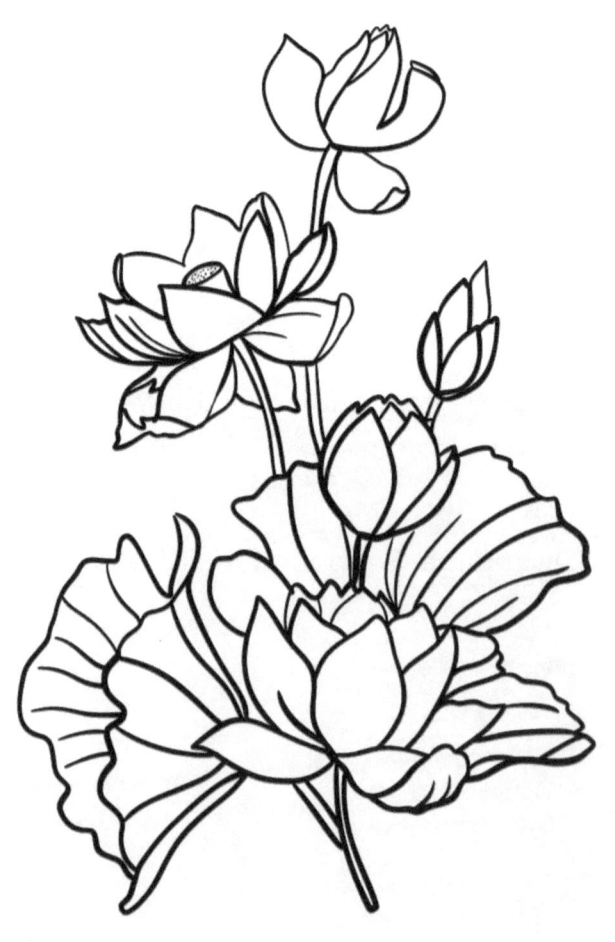

CHAPTER FIFTEEN

Cult

Rest

Let's venture into the truest part of ourselves in this chapter's resting practice. The meditation is waiting for you on youreenoughyoga.com.

Recovery

What matters the most to you in your life? What would your life be like if you had greater levels of self-confidence, self-esteem or more love in your life? Imagine you have all of these things along with the time to focus on what matters to you. Picture your life with you being successful, breaking through your perceived constraints and limitations. Are you creating big things in your life, or do you want to see positive change in the world? Do you have goals to reach extraordinary levels of success or just a niggling feeling that surely there is more to life? If this is you, welcome to the next step of your life as you begin your journey with Olympus Seminars.

Inspiring pitch? It is exactly the kind of language that seems to see inside a person's thoughts, language that helps a person feel seen, understood and full of world-changing potential.

Millions of people worldwide are participating in programs with Olympus Seminars, from CEOs, athletes, scientists, students to stay-at-home parents. These participants report exponential growth across the board in their lives, with major results in the areas of relationships, finance and career. Participants experience a deeper connection with their life's purpose thanks to the process used in Olympus's programs.

Sound convincing or like a bunch of word-salad, over-reaching cliches?

Your life is happening right now, every moment passing by. Will you stay daydreaming about your goals or take action right now to begin living a powerful, fulfilling life? Look, things may be OK in your life now, but what else is possible for you? Stop wondering if you will ever be good enough, stop putting it off and do something amazing for yourself. Take out the form from your leaflet and book your Olympus weekend now.

The Hook

I wanted to be good enough. How did they know that this was my problem, always feeling like I didn't belong, sometimes believing I was too much for people, but mostly feeling I was simply not enough? I hugged my friend who had invited me to this open evening at Olympus Seminars (not this cult's real name), took out the little white card from inside the leaflet, hurriedly filled it in and rushed over to one of the registration tables. In black pen, I filled in the flimsy credit card slip with my details and handed it over to the total stranger behind the grey desk. *Old school*, I thought, *no credit card machines.*

I have ruminated on and replayed this moment zillions of times. Watching it play in my memory as my late thirties self, I want to teleport into that exact moment when the credit card slip was still in my 24-year-old self's hand, calmly take it away from younger Sarah and tear it up. Linking arms with her, I would get our coats and say,

'Give it a miss, babe. There is nothing for you here.'

Off we would stroll into the warm evening.

You might have guessed that, in actual fact, I did not stroll off into the summer's evening. Instead, I paid a £50 deposit to book my spot in a weekend 'course' which was touted as personal development combined with an enquiry into the nature of being human. It sounded fascinating to me. I had always been a searcher, voracious to understand the weirdness of being human ever since I said no to religious

Sunday school at age seven. I was convinced that being alive was more complex than what had been written about a man called God by some ancient dead men thousands of years ago. I was also relatively new in town, and I was looking for like-minded people to hang out with. The weekend course sounded perfect for me.

Human beings have always wanted to improve themselves and have a deeper understanding of why we are all here on this blue and green planet. People want to know the meaning of life. Surely there must be more to my experience of being human than the outdated corrupt system that I live in? Is this the only reality? There is nothing wrong with pondering these questions that have bugged humans from time immemorial. Many spiritual traditions such as Yoga, Eastern Tantra, Gnosticism and, more recently, Reiki explore the essential practice of connecting us humans with our original, spiritual nature as fractals of the Universe. The quest for personal growth and self-development is often the portal many seekers like myself step through before these larger, more head-spinning kinds of ponderings about our place in the Universe and connection to all beings start to reveal themselves.

The problem is that the fundamental desire for self-improvement is the entry level or metaphorical shop window to deceive and entice people through a cult's shiny, spinning glass doors and marbled entrance halls. The next minute you're hearing the hard sell, which encourages participants to act right now to buy course after course, inevitably taking participants closer to the toxic centre of these organisations, deeper into indoctrination and the tiptoe into being abused by the high-demand group (cultic group) similar to the ones I found myself in. These cults that lure people with glossy guarantees of self-improvement and more confidence may focus around personal development, group therapy, business mentoring, multi-level marketing, spirituality, modern mystery schools, yoga, and tantra, to name but a few types of content that cults use to scam and abuse people.

Let's take a beat here so I can myth-bust. Think you are too clever/alert/sceptical to get drawn into a cultic organisation? I definitely thought I would be able to spot a cult coming for me a mile off! Turns out I couldn't, because every person who is not in a coma is vulnerable to mind control techniques and indoctrination. Everybody is susceptible to the love-bombing, manipulation, loaded language, thought stopping, coercion and duplicity enacted by charismatic leaders and the cult followers whom they collect to do their bidding. We are all susceptible to the undue influence which cults bear over the lives and minds of their members. If I asked you if you wanted to join a group which would definitely abuse you in these ways, I'm guessing you would either politely decline or ask me if I had lost my shit. The thing is, nobody knowingly joins a group that will harm them; people sign up for courses and retreats that they have been manipulated to believe will benefit them. People want to join groups which promise to offer all the answers to life's complexities, which promise a sense of community and hope through the realisation of the group's grandiose promises. Let's be real though, no group, religion or person has ALL the answers. Communities can be turned into emotionally toxic environments and hope can be used to manipulate members to stay in a group to prove their beliefs and test their loyalty. You probably wouldn't want to join a group where this is the hidden reality. Of course you wouldn't, because it is a scam.

Ending up in a cult is not the survivor's fault and nothing to be ashamed of. Mic drop.

Cults Feed on the Curse of Not Enough

While everybody is vulnerable to the psychological abuse carried out by cults, from my personal experience on the inside, hearing the stories of people who have stayed in the group I joined and those who have thankfully left, along with research into other cult recruitment techniques, there is a theme. I signed up to the course they offered because I thought I was fundamentally flawed, while I was also incredibly motivated to improve myself. I was a cult recruiter's dream! I thought I was not a good enough woman, thanks to patriarchal society. I did not feel at home with who I was, and I just wanted to believe that I was OK. I thought I needed to be more go-getting but also more chilled, more confident and less emotional, so I could save my then boyfriend from my anxiety and tears. I was scared I was driving him crazy because he had said numerous times that I was too emotional. I believed I needed to get a handle on myself, put a lid on what he called my 'negativity'. This negativity was, in fact, a set of mental health issues all under the umbrella of an eating disorder. I did not need to be going to preachy, ass-kicking, fervour-inducing large group seminars. What I needed was care, empathy, and medical intervention for my illness. But my shame towards my 'too much' emotions coupled with my core belief that I was not good enough drew me towards abusive organisations, which mirrored my own unconscious habit of abusing myself. I would hear similar stories to mine time and again from women I was tasked to recruit while I worked in the sales departments of the organisations I was duped into; *I need to believe in myself more, I think I'm failing at my life, I need to get promoted, I want to know how to attract a man.* Women who believed that something was wrong about them, and they needed somebody or something to fix them. Truthfully, I would hear the male versions of the 'not good enough' beliefs too; *I need to get to the next level in my career so I can impress my parents, I want to find a super hot girlfriend because all my mates have that, I need to learn how to be more positive, to stop letting my emotions slow me down.*

I took my first 'course' in the early 2000s. A wave of nausea just came over me as I typed that date. I had to pause to soothe and send Reiki to the ache in the pit of my abdomen, my womb space. This was clearly a message from myself to myself that my body remembers the accumulated stress of being around this organisation for four years. This course marked the gateway into four years of being subtly and not so subtly mind controlled, being coaxed into believing I would fail at life without the organisation and their 'training', of overriding and gradually losing my trust in myself and my body's wisdom. This cult is damaging to anybody who stays around long enough to get sucked in, but I am absolutely clear that the ultimate damage I endured during my time there was the eroding of any felt sense of my Feminine nature.

The organisation was not patriarchal in the sense that there was any explicit favouring of men over women; the patriarchal aroma was more subtle than that. However, during the time that I worked there, this aroma became a foul stench the closer I got to the inner circle of senior leadership. Both men and women were in the upper echelons of the group's hierarchy, and during my time working there in a paid role (thousands of people do unpaid work within this group, a sure sign of a high-demand group), I often took direction and what was termed 'coaching' from women in superior roles to mine. I would be coached so that I could handle any lack of performance around my sales role. The underlying vibe of this coaching was getting me to reject my connection with anything other than what I needed to do to perform. In this case, performance meant how many seats in a course I could sell. This target was micromanaged through to how many sales calls I could make every hour. I needed to submit my results to my manager every two hours so that she could check that I was keeping my targets and daily sales results. If I had missed my target/result, coaching would occur to see what my problem was that I wasn't delivering the sales results they pressured me to produce. The coaching told me that it was always my fault. I now understand that this 'coaching' was in fact mind control to keep me obedient. After all these years away from the group I still have an aversion to the word 'coach' and all things coaching!

Let's break this down against the context of the whole organisation: the sales environment in the cult echoed the teachings of its seminars, in short, that there is zero reason not to perform at a high level all the time, and I mean all the damn time. No justifications, no explanations, no reasons. Anything that a participant thought was a reasonable obstacle to their ability to produce results in their life was just an excuse or an example of their constrained, small thinking. You see, in this place, everything had to be big and bold all the time. There was no place for subtlety, ebbs and flows, the inevitability that life sometimes goes one step forward and two steps back and this is not a reflection on the individual's abilities or intrinsic worth. Example:

You want to be in the relationship of your dreams in the next six months. Promise it to your course leader or coach. What actions you will take every day to produce this result. How many dates do you promise to go on each week to fulfil on this result? Not had a date this week? Do you care more about feeling sorry for yourself and staying single or actually achieving results? Or: You want to lose that weight. How many minutes of exercise do you promise every day? Tell your coach so they can keep you accountable (this meant text/call you all the time to check what you are up to). Not done your exercise this week? You clearly are not committed to improving your fitness but you are committed to your excuses.

There is so much to unpack in this example, all of it with a flavour of undue influence. The abusive system of this organisation was focused on pressing participants to keeping their word by delivering results – intensely praising the participant in a short burst of attention if they kept their word, then immediately pressing them to set and achieve the next big goal without any time to regroup, rest, reflect and nourish oneself. Course participants and staff were influenced not to think, but to always be taking action. It was a stressful environment because everything was portrayed as urgent. Predictably, as is the hallmark of cults, the next big goal would only be achievable upon paying for the next program run by the group. If the participant did not achieve their stated goal, then they would be invalidated as per the loaded question in the above example and forced to admit the reason for their lack of success. The coach or course leader, with zero empathy, would deconstruct the participant's insights into an excuse.

What passed for coaching in the culture of this group, from my own experience of being coached both as a participant and staff member along with coaching I was trained to give course participants, was more like harsh, coerced confession time. The coachee would be encouraged to look back into their life and revisit some painful memory which might be stopping them from living their best life. Participants were encouraged to share private information about themselves, which was often traumatic for them to revisit. Inevitably, it would be implied by the leader or coach that their emotional pain was more important to them than their goal and not a valid reason for failing to manifest the results they wanted in their life. Yep, vomit. I was trained to do this by the group, and I could not see that this methodology was abusive. I had some serious shame about behaving in this way toward people. Neither could I see that this organisation, supposedly based on empowerment, was in fact a cult whose goal was to get people in and keep them in.

Patriarchy loves high production, which is achieved by single-mindedness employed to relentlessly pursue a forced result. Imagine a male, cane-wielding, moustachioed Soviet factory boss from an Orwellian nightmare, ready to beat his workers if not enough potatoes are packed per hour. This is the unbalanced masculine blueprint for approaching life: find it, chase it, get it, squeeze out what you want from it, no matter what. This version of Masculinity has been promoted by patriarchy as a means to an end for perpetuating itself as an oppressive force upon all things Feminine. Being in this cult felt like I was being monitored by an invisible, threatening, cane-wielding force day in and day out. It was utterly draining and unsustainable. Other women who have left the inner circles (paid staff and senior level course leaders) of this organisation have shared with me that they were left exhausted, ill from the fear of not producing the results they were pressed for. I am still deprogramming from the overly productive, unforgiving all-masculine way of living that was promoted by this group.

Starving

When I finally left, I was vulnerable, confused, exhausted and starving for the Feminine. Four years on an emotional rollercoaster induced by the back-to-front, upside-down doublethink of a cult really fucked with my mind and body. It is ironic that this emotional roller coaster was caused by a cult which teaches that feelings (particularly those aching, intuitive gut feelings) were not something worth bothering with. Part of the manipulation used by the group persuaded women members to ignore our emotions, to override the pain in our bodies caused by overwork (it's all in your head!) and pretend we did not need regular rest. The coaching for all staff to produce results on the hour every hour caused me so much distress that I would head to the bathrooms and cry. Literally, I would run because the fear of time away from working at my desk and missing my target caused my body to move fast and frantically. I was traumatised. The organisation thrived off the unhealthy aspects of toxic masculine work ethic and leadership. There was no healthy Masculine here, the supportive Masculine energy which holds space for and wants to serve Feminine energy so that She may move with Her cycles, brewing, creating and birthing accordingly. Whatever I did there, it would never be enough for them; that much is true, but because of their unrelenting press for results and encouragement to abandon a healthy sense of self, I was indoctrinated to believe that I was not good enough. Not only not good enough but too much, wayward if my results did not improve quick-sharp. I was told that I deliberately, wilfully failed at my job so I could be destructive. WHAT??? This frequent gaslighting meant that I struggled to keep a grip on my reality. I remember one of the higher-ups apoplectically raging at me one day when nobody had booked the course I was selling. To paraphrase:

'If you refuse to perform then you can just get the fuck out.'

One of the junior members asked if I was OK. I pretended it was all in jest, but on the inside, I was terrified and in shock. I wish I had got my coat and just fucked off but I had been trained to be obedient.

The reality was that I was being disconnected from my inner sense of safety, struggling to hear my Feminine wisdom telling me that I was being abused by a covertly patriarchal system.

Abusing the Feminine

You see, life goes well when we balance structured, action-oriented commitments, which are intrinsic to Masculine energy, with cyclical, creative, feeling-centred, introspective subtleties intrinsic to Feminine energy. Back to the earlier example of a person who wants to lose weight:

You want to lose some weight. What kind of exercise feels good for you, what movement do you enjoy? What would be an inviting amount of movement you could work toward each week? Listen to your body's needs so you can be compassionate to yourself if you need to skip a day if you feel unwell or want to rest on your period. Do you have somebody you feel comfortable with who could support your ongoing fitness journey if you ask for some encouragement?

How does this example feel compared with the first iteration of coaching to lose weight? It is a combination of Masculine and Feminine approaches: action and structure combined with compassion for the body's cyclical needs. This is the type of guidance that helps a person stay connected with their own wisdom rather than overriding one's needs in favour of smashing out a result of the patriarchal, production-driven, no matter what vibe.

Let's remember, though, that cults abuse people whether they rely on singularly Masculine-style or purely Feminine-inspired teachings, or both. The content of a cult is irrelevant because what damages people is the systematic erosion of one's self-worth, the essential connection with and belief in our enoughness, that we will be just fine without the group's supposed pearls of wisdom. A sure sign of cultic dynamics from a group or individual is any implication that your life won't be as enjoyable/successful/fulfilling/whole without them. Both of the cultic organisations I survived dined out on this fallacy – the premise that you need to belong to the group to be happy, that they are the only ones who know and appreciate you and only they are the ones who have the answers you seek. When a person hears this manipulation frequently, or it is implied strongly again and again over an extended time, the person in the cult will favour this lie. I used to listen to it as truth over and above my own spidey-sense or inner voice saying that something was off, and ignore the uneasy lurching of my tummy when I entered my office at Cult HQ. My body was showing me every day that something was indeed amiss, toxic, dangerous. This severing of the connection between mind and body is an attack, an abuse upon the Feminine. The Feminine is the subtlety of body sensation, the niggles that niggle us in gut feelings, the wisdom to pause and say, 'NO, what is happening here is wrong'. Cults try to destroy women's ability to listen to themselves, the cues from our bodies, even the cults which pride themselves on female empowerment. It is toxic power dynamics 101 and patriarchy loves itself some toxic power.

I harboured A LOT of anger towards this organisation, which is rotten at its core, but I never felt anger toward my immediate colleagues. These are brilliant, warm, committed people who, like me, thought they were changing the world.

BITE Me

I was in and out of two cults for about six years. Cult A promised an Incredible Life and Cult B told me that I would learn how to be an Irresistible Woman. There has been a lot of unlearning and recovering from the harm done to me. During those six years, I returned twice to Cult A, which focused on personal development via large-group awareness training. During my time working there, I became incredibly sick with horrendous stress-related migraines to the point where I would suffer temporary one-sided paralysis due to this condition called 'migraine with aura'. My body knew that something was deeply wrong, and manifested this as physical illness. I was off work for a month or so, but still within the control of the cultic antics. They called me every day and told me that my recovery was too slow, adding that I was not 'causing' my recovery. That is one of the many problems with cults; they make out that you are deficient at everything. On one of these long manipulative calls, one of the bosses said to me:

'You're just chicken shit.'

That was enough. I sent in my resignation that same week. I quit working there and stayed away for a couple of years, and, of course, my migraines stopped, and I got stronger, but I had not fully accepted that I had been duped and emotionally abused by this organisation. I returned to the courses a couple of years later. I was in a very low place and was recovering from being raped. I wanted that influx of positive energy whipped up by the group's courses, the fervour which had sucked me right in that first time. This just shows how hard it is to totally extricate from any kind of abusive relationship, particularly this relationship with the group I had invested years of my life in. Thankfully, I left for good around seven years after joining.

Cult A professed that it wanted to empower people to be in love with their lives. My experience as a woman in this organisation was one of being coerced out of my Femininity and into being an obedient, corporate, emotion-dodging, harsh, gaslighted, cold, exhausted droid who was indoctrinated to believe my life would be a shit show without them. That's what they do: make members think they are not enough without the group. My life was a shit show WITH them and gradually became bloody ace without them. Cult B has been under investigation by the FBI for sex trafficking. 'Nuff said.

What both of these groups have in common are the abuse tactics which are what makes a cult. This criteria for recognising abuse in a high demand group/cult is called the BITE Model and it's the work of ex-cult-member and cult expert Steven Hassan.[1] The BITE model includes behaviour control, information control, thought control and emotion control. The tactics also feature in any coercively controlling relationship. Cult A and B feature fuckloads of these tactics, too many to list in this book, but here is a flavour:

Behaviour Control

Cult A banned staff and leaders from engaging in any other personal growth courses or modalities outside of Cult A.

Cult B coerced members to pursue sexual contact with people they did not find attractive, as a method of overcoming the supposed binds of personal preference.

Information Control

Staff and leaders at Cult A were given a list of Corporate Answers to learn as responses to any questions we were ever asked by lower-ranking members or non-members. We were tested on these answers to make sure we represented Cult A the way it wanted to be perceived – for example, as not being a cult!

Cult B kept sensitive information about course participants on spreadsheets e.g., *struggles to connect with women*, so that the sales team could use this as intelligence and guide manipulatory sales conversations.

Thought Control

We were told to always be vigilant about our thoughts; mindfuck.

Cult A wanted staff and leaders to be in constant communication to their manager and report any thoughts they were having that could hinder their sales performance. For example, thoughts about being tired or thoughts doubting you should call this person for a fourth time to see if they wanted to register for a course yet. On reporting these thoughts, we were told to make a more empowering thought.

Cult B would run an exercise where the coach would ask endless questions to a participant. The answers were the participant's private thoughts which they were encouraged to share so they could 'keep their lines clean'. Yeah, sorry for the word salad; cults are full of bizarre language.

Emotion Control

Cult A had a total disregard for emotion. Emotions were apparently our excuses for our poor performance. However, because we were coached so harshly by upper management, inevitably people would break down in tears on the regular, which made for a poisonous work environment. On crying, this was invalidated, and a person would be reminded by a coach or manager that this was behaviour of a junior course graduate, not a leader.

They also used fear and threats to control us. I was threatened that I would not get my full monthly wages if I did not register enough people into courses. My wages were never meant to be performance related.

Cult B – When I was sexually assaulted at a music festival, having taken a weekend away from cult activities, one leader told me this was the kind of thing that happens when you go away. What a way to victim-blame! I was made to feel guilty for going away and fearful of the outside world – correction, even *more* fearful, as I was already traumatised by the assault.

Cult A and Cult B feature on many online search results for lists of recognised cults. Cult A asserts informational control by strongly suggesting that new and long-term members do not read these online analyses! I am not naming these cults because, frankly, I do not have the money to hire a lawyer if they decided to sue me or go after the publisher! That's just another trick from the cult playbook: litigate and financially abuse till kingdom come.

If you think you may have accidentally got caught up with a demanding group or recognise cultic traits in a group you are in, and you want to give them the heave-ho, then I salute you for listening to that crucial gut feeling. That is your Feminine energy talking to you. There is a list of resources that you might find helpful for your deprogramming and healing at the back of this book.

Rising

Have you ever felt stuck in a situation you felt you could not leave?

What did your gut instinct tell you about the situation?

Journal, draw or collage on the word 'belonging'. What does it mean to you?

Does the rational portion of your brain win above your gut feelings, or vice versa?

With reference to patriarchy (including religion, politics, and institutions) do you recognise any examples of behaviour control, information control, thought control and emotional control?

How might you begin to untangle from these four examples of mind control which are inflicted by patriarchy?

All cults have something in common, as well as training people to believe they are not enough outside of the grip of the cult. Cults thrive on the abuse of power. We will dive into the system's obsession with power at all costs and the impact this has upon women during the next chapter. But let's take a breather first.

Take Your Power Back.

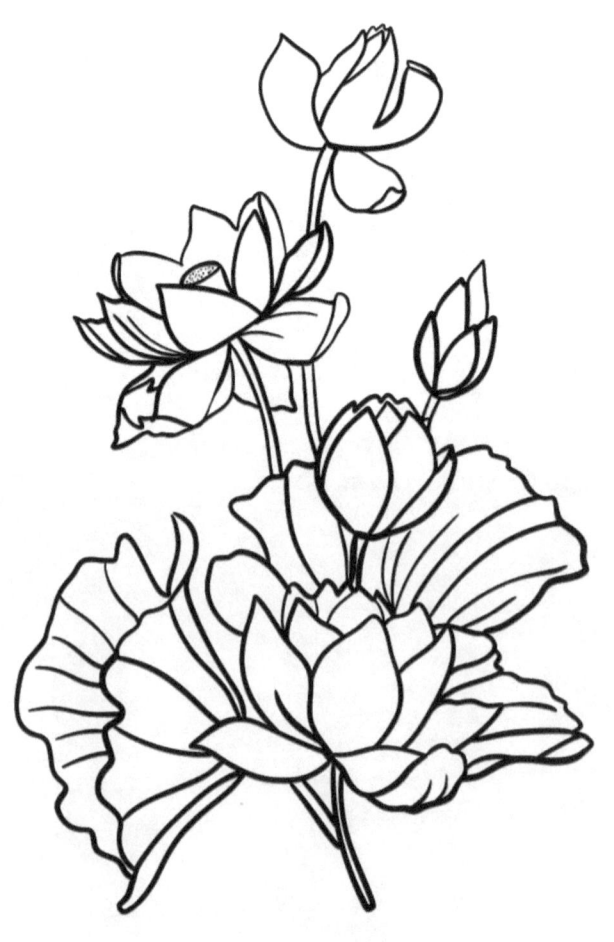

CHAPTER SIXTEEN

Power

Rest

It's time for some silence. Glide over to the Enough! area on my website for your resting meditation.

Recovery

> 'From this hour on, for the time of the due
> season of the aeon, I will receive rest in silence.'
> – Mary 9:29

What comes to mind when you read the word 'power'? Sit quietly for a few minutes and journal or doodle your ideas. What came through? My mind turns to patriarchy, of course! Along with politicians abusing power, discrimination, religion, Big Brother embodied from Orwell's writing, scandal, lies, conspiracy and autonomy.

Questions about power have pervaded the woman-psyche for thousands of years: what does it mean to be in our power? How would we act if we embodied our power? Do women or men have the power? If patriarchy has vowed to restrict the rights and voices of women, is this because they know our power? What about the questions of race, womanhood and power? Do women of colour societally lose out in favour of white women? Definitely, that is the beast of white supremacy. I believe that so much of our experience of womanhood and our experiences of enoughness are bound up with our relationship to power. Frankly, it feels like patriarchy's curse of too much and not enough is a power play to disconnect women from their power; from the parts of us that know deep inside our hearts that we are enough, the inner voice that tells us that society is wrong, and not us who are fundamentally flawed for not living up to Superwoman standards, day in and day out. Go back as far as the suppression of pagan Goddess worship by the early Church and the suppression of reverence for the Feminine face of God as understood in Gnosticism, and we see the pattern of power being stolen from women, along with the opportunity for anyone to venerate the potency of Feminine energy.

What has changed? Tell a religious person (not including pagans) that you believe Feminine power is the ultimate power or that God could have a Feminine side as well as the Masculine aspect, and get ready to see their eyes glaze over as they smile and nod while deep down they wish they were getting to work casting the demon out of you. Tell a fundamentalist believer from any Abrahamic religion that you have an inkling that there may not be a male God but rather a Universal Life Force which is Feminine, and they are likely to advise you to pray for God's (the male one's!) forgiveness for such bad thoughts or start damming you to Hell for this heretical transgression! Patriarchal religion has so much to answer for because many of the world's women are oppressed under varying abusive fundamentalist religious regimes that purport that God is male and ONLY male. Therefore, it is a no-brainer that men need to hold more power than women while women must endure being oppressed under the guise of being told that they are serving God through these restraints. Religious fundamentalists gaslight women by dressing up oppression and abuse of women as being for their own good. They say there must be gender-based rules on women so that they do not tempt the pious males to sin by looking at women. It is crazy-making that women are shown that they do not deserve any power, which teaches them they are not enough, not worthy of power, but at the same time, rules about conduct infer that women are powerful enough to cause a man to sin if women, for example, (Goddess-forbid) dress immodestly.

As I have already noted, conveying women as the problem which could tempt men into bad or un-Godly behaviour is all part of patriarchy's game of too much and not enough. In Fundamentalist Hasidic Jewish communities teenage boys are discouraged from speaking to their female peers in the street just in case this causes the boy to have thoughts about the girl that God would not approve of, e.g., feeling attracted to the girl or enjoying her company, which would surely lead the young chap into a whole world of transgression and, as a result, falling out of favour with God. In other words, this boy's fall from God's grace would be the fault of the girl for triggering the interest from the boy. If we break this down again it seems as if the boys of this fundamentalist community are believed to be deserving of protection from girls, while girls must suffer the trauma of arranged teenage marriage, the indignity of untold amounts of household toil, and no sex education.

Something Rotten

Fundamentalist religion personifies the confusing relationship to power which all women must navigate. Sure, not every woman grows up in fundamentalist religious communities which are blatant and shameless in their suppression of women, but the power that is asserted over women in secular society is also confusing and damaging. We only need consider society's discriminatory and misogynist treatment of menopausal women to see that something is deeply rotten inside the power structures of businesses and institutions. In a 2021 *Guardian* feature, a handful of women spoke out about the abhorrent treatment doled out to them inside their workplace cultures when they were cycling through menopause symptoms.[1] One woman detailed the constant pressure of weekly performance reviews and the looming warnings of being fired, as a measure to increase her performance, having been told by management she was underperforming while under the stress of severe menopause symptoms: brain fog, depression, sweats, and joint pain. Another woman was marginalised while training to be in the police service, a trainer pointing her out in front of peers as a 'bloody knackered menopausal woman'. I've no idea the gender of this trainer but it doesn't matter, it's still shitty and unacceptable, I just hope it was not a female doling out this abuse because it would be even more vile coming from a woman. The trainee's colleague explained, 'That's just how it is here. You won't get anywhere,' following the police service's HR department stonewalling her complaints. Culturally, Western patriarchy treats our wise and valuable women like shit, when, in fact, menopausal women deserve maximum respect for the wisdom and power they are coming to possess in the process of menopause. The toxic power of patriarchy cares not for the inclusion of women's wellbeing. Women who will continue to offer valuable skills and experience to the workplace until whenever the woman sees fit to retire, which if you live in the good ol' U S of A will be far into old age because of that system's refusal to offer good wages for all workers or salient pension options.

We Women Are the Power

Misogyny attempts to assert power over women behind closed doors as well as in wider society's blatant displays in the examples above. I recognise how it feels to walk on eggshells, feeling prickly and anxious that I may say the wrong thing, which would expose me as being too much or not good enough. I had a male partner once who would not let me stay in the room with him if I ever cried; he would say I was a female stereotype who was unskilled in dealing with her emotions. For him, dealing with emotions meant suppressing emotions. My experience in this relationship made me feel dehumanised and invalidated. In a screwed-up way, I believed I deserved this invalidation because I messed up all the time by showing emotion, and I did not want to upset this man by being too much. If I had any hope of keeping this dude on the scene then I needed to get better at being the type of woman I was being moulded into. Of course, after years of therapy to help me heal from the toxic power dynamics inflicted by my closest relationships, I know that suppressing my 'too much' emotions was not helpful for me, but only enabled the pattern of misogynist abuse present in that relationship. You have no idea how much I wish to bump into that man who was intent on asserting societally enabled patriarchal control over me, and telling him to go fuck himself. I'm sure he'd just love being accosted by my overly emotional female stereotype that he was so repulsed by in our unhealthy relationship! Nah, fuck it, he's not worth it because abusers like him deserve zero attention.

We know by now that the roots of patriarchy robbing women of power and freedom is due to people clinging to the belief that God, the supposedly all-seeing, all-knowing, all-powerful chap, is male. Vis a vis, the male of the species should have more power or be viewed as more important and influential than women. Jesus, that last sentence taken out of context reads like a line from a fundamentalist Christian pamphlet! I feel grimy just thinking about the fact that some people really believe that being shitty toward women, imposing this confusing fog that causes us to question whether we are enough or too much or both, is fine and dandy because they can defend their unhealthy power plays on religious grounds. I totally just took some time out to ground myself with a Yoga Nidrā practice to avoid my brain exploding with indignation!

Conspiracy

The historical fixation with male God = male power has resulted in the wilful conspiracy to suppress the work and spiritual teachings of, in my humble opinion, one of the world's most underrated and misrepresented female spiritual teachers. She was co-existing and co-working with Jesus while nurturing her own spiritual community based upon the love and compassion that exist in everyone. Sounds a bit hippy-trippy-peace and love? OK, yes, love and compassion do not exist in all people because there are psychopaths, sociopaths, and malignant narcissists who wreak havoc on this planet. The modern world has become a playground for those who wish to dominate power over others. Light and love do not flow from these folks, and we need to disengage and set boundaries to protect ourselves from those who seek to abuse power. That being said, I do trust that there are truckloads of love inside the majority of people who do not pathologically act out vindictive, harmful patterns.

This woman's teachings were part of a set of teachings recorded by hand and literally buried in the Egyptian desert. Their burial may echo the rationale for suppressing the material found on these buried scrolls. These scrolls, which have come to be known as the Nag Hammadi texts or the Gnostic Gospels, speak to a style of Christianity which was not accepted by the fathers of the early Church. This early version of Christianity was called Gnosticism and purported that every human has a spark of divine (or, Godly) intelligence within. Some call this spark pure love, and with this loving intelligence, we can experience the divine while down here on planet Earth. The Gnostics believed humans were already empowered with the gnosis (knowledge) that we have something in common with God and the Universe, an inner divinity or deep love residing in us. This connection to God meant that humans did not have to search far for a source of benevolent power; it was already within. These beliefs did not fit with the teachings of the fathers of the early Church, who proselytised that there was a God who was very separate from humans and that we are ultimately under His control. The possibility that humans had a direct, non-hierarchical relationship with the loving creator spirit plus a glimmer of that source within us would have meant that the Church was not all-powerful in delivering the word of God as they propagandised it, nor could they control people who listened to their own wisdom rather than only believing they were at the mercy of God. The Gnostics did not need to be part of the Church to commune with God. Through trance, they could tap into the feelings of love and creativity already born into them and hear their own wisdom as to how to conduct themselves. No Church dogma necessary!

The scrolls found at Nag Hammadi contained metaphysical writings examining the nature of consciousness and the link between mind and matter, the formless and form. These musings were unpopular, to say the least, with the leaders of the first iterations of the organised Church because the authors of these texts were mulling over ideas which suggested we humans are divine and have this divinity in common with God. As if that were not scandalous enough, what about a possibility that there is not one all-powerful male God, but possibly an original Feminine creator of our universe who we can feel when we connect with the love that lives inside us?

The jury is still out on the definite reason for the scrolls being buried. I bet it has to do with early Christians wanting to save these documents that had been branded heresy and, under Church law in AD 367, were deemed illegal because they were not on the approved religious reading list stipulated by the Bishop of Alexandria. Like I said, having the teachings of a woman recorded on scrolls for all to see would have been a spanner in the works of the Church's mission to deny the possibility of an originating, Feminine creative force. The name of this divine Feminine force, or Goddess, is Sophia. Gnostic writings and beliefs tell a tale of how Mother Earth and everything in her were formed from Sophia's formless state as she descended from a nebula way out in space. Notice that this is a very different creation story from the biblical telling of a chap named God making the Earth in seven days! Sophia's myth feels right to me. For the emerging patriarchy, it was too much to fathom that a Feminine force birthed our universe into existence. It just did not fit the rollout of the control measures to eradicate any belief systems, such as Gnosticism and paganism, which did not echo the one-size-fits-all narrative of the one and only powerful male God. This woman, who not only spoke her truth of powerful divine love within humans but also dared to teach her truth, became prey to a smear campaign against her enforced by patriarchy. I was taught the lies about her when I was a child before I made my sharp exit from those weekly Sunday school sessions.

I Heart Mary

Mary Magdalene was not a prostitute. Mary Magdalene was a teacher who instructed people to go beyond the layers of personality and fears which separate us from our divinity. She teaches us to consciously spend time connecting with the force of love inside, the love that rests deep in the cave of our heart, and in this place, we find the power of the divine Feminine. If you think this is all sounding rather *Da Vinci Code*, then you are right! Dan Brown dined out on the myth of Mary Magdalene in his popular novel. He added a fair bit of artistic licence by suggesting that Mary's entombed body is, in fact, the Holy Grail hidden for protection by the Knights Templar (sorry, spoiler if you are one of the few people who has not read the novel or enjoyed Tom Hanks rushing around London's sacred sites in the film adaptation!) from the evil Catholic sect Opus Dei. Unsurprisingly, I'm not well versed with the secretive Opus Dei, who are portrayed as a group of fundamentalist, self-flagellating, robe-wearing old blokes in Brown's novel. However, I am familiar with stories that the Church has tried to keep the wisdom of Mary's gospel under wraps, along with the possibility that she bore Jesus's daughter during her exile in the South of France. Scandalous – I love it.

The message of Mary's gospel is clear: love. Thanks to Feminist Theologian Meggan Watterson's exploration of Mary Magdalene's teachings, I began to understand that Mary was a proponent of the inner wisdom or gnosis that resides inside us. She did not want people to place their only notion of power upon an entity called God somewhere in the heavens, or on forces outside ourselves, but instead to turn our focus inward so we can lean into the well of love, wisdom, and power which has been with us all along. Mary wants us to get quiet, to meditate, to hear the benevolent power of our highest selves for our highest good, rather than chasing the short-term gratifications of power as lapped up by the ego. I resonate with the message and the all-important reminder from Watterson that this is no quick fix but a practice to repeat 'again and again'. If I had a pound for every time I had turned to something outside of myself, be it a man, booze, drugs, sex, exercise, food (or lack of it), or social media validation to give me a fleeting feeling of okayness, enoughness, worthiness, damn it even a misplaced sense of power, then I would be rich as fuck.

Anyone Seen My Power?

My searching in people, places, and things for my own enoughness, my own power, is the textbook behaviour of addiction. The driver of the behaviour is the sense of disconnection from or emptiness of one's own self-worth. I used to have a gaping hole in my enoughness well, and this inability to love myself used to trick me into searching for my worth in all the wrong places.

'I just don't understand what is wrong with me! Why does this keep happening? I can't deal with this again.'

I was recovering from an unexpected, very sudden break-up. As was my pattern – as I have come to understand it, thanks to much self-reflection, meditation and skilful therapists(!) – I had quickly flung every bit of me into a relationship with a dude who was a toxic blend of incredibly exciting, attentive, suave, and emotionally illiterate. I thought we were falling in love, but my thoughts about us were mixed up. I figured that I must be enough because I was dating him, and somebody like him would only date somebody he deemed good enough. Yet I had increasingly loud, frequent thoughts that he would leave me because he would find somebody better, as I would not be able to sustain my levels of good enough for long enough. Round and round my mind circled on this exhausting carousel. My efforts to please him while making it look like it was all effortless were no match for my inner wounding, my belief that I was not enough.

There was no row, no argument, it was simple. One day we were together, the next day his ghosting began. This was the latest of my relationships to end up like this; he's here one day, puff, vanished the next.

'You're not quite what I'm looking for,' read the text he sent me four days later.

Out of nowhere, I heaved to throw up. What was it this time? Was I not enough or too much, or both?

Honestly, the couple of weeks after that text are blurry. I went to my first Love and Sex Addicts Anonymous meeting when I eventually felt more human.

'Hi, I'm Sarah and I think I might be a love addict. Somebody said I should come here and listen.'

Leaning into Love

I only attended a handful of meetings. The unbending, formulaic structure of the meetings and the hierarchy of sponsors and sponsees did not feel great, but the space was welcoming. Plus, I think I heard the piece of the puzzle which I needed during that first meeting. I heard a theme in people's sharing: *emptiness, hungry, something missing, self-care, need to know who I am, want to believe I am worth it, stop looking outside myself.* I was learning that it was not just me who needed to fill up on the transient pleasures of relationships, drink, and drugs. In this dingy room downstairs in the belly of a church, the walls cold and slightly damp, cave-like, I heard my own and other people's humanity speak: pain, rejection, confusion, lust, chasing, romance, abandonment, yearning, empathy, hope. Everything that makes us wholly human and, as Mary Magdalene would have us believe, wholly divine. I felt my heart speak to me as I wandered through the dusky, ivy-entangled graveyard in central London. I heard my quiet voice of self-compassion, the will to fight to bring myself back from the edge, the knowledge that I am not wrong for being who I am. The rescue I sought to find in partners would come from me instead. I resolved to learn to love myself. It has been messy, painful, thrilling, nourishing and very, very human. I uncovered my enoughness within quiet meditation, writing about my pain in words that nobody will ever see, medication when I needed it, nourishing my body with the right food, right movement and rest, with the grace and dissolution of Yoga Nidrā, the stillness and flow of yoga asana, the decoded teachings of Mary Magdalene that my power rests in the repetition of leaning back into my own wellspring of love. Enoughness is within. As Meggan Watterson says in her book *Mary Magdalene Revealed*, 'Love is within us. We do not have to earn or prove or deserve this fact' and that, my friend, is power. Feminine power.

Drumroll, Please ... Introducing a Voice of Power and Wisdom

What I've explored so far in this chapter is just one alternative embodiment of power which contrasts with patriarchy's version of power as oppression, suppression, a power over others. While exploring my own ideas about how power is expressed by men versus women, Masculine versus Feminine, healthy versus unhealthy power, it occurred to me that I had more questions than answers! I needed the help of a wise woman (who so does not relate to herself as an expert, but she totally is!) versed in both Western and Eastern spiritual paths to help me untangle my questions about power. My chat with the wise woman Cathy Rowan lifted the veil to reveal a new face of Feminine power which is still blowing my mind months after our long Zoom chat. This is what Cathy is saying about the style of power expressed in Femininity and Masculinity, patriarchy's dirty tricks of too much and not enough and the true power of the Feminine:

Me: Cathy, in your own words how would you define Feminine power?

Cathy: Firstly, let's start with defining the term Feminine because it is used in different ways. There is the one level where we use the word Feminine to talk about attributes of gender. The other way that this term Feminine is used is in psychological terms, regarding inner qualities such as the inner Feminine or inner Masculine, and these days we often speak about Feminine energy and Masculine energy, which are held by each person no matter their gender. This can relate to opposites like Yin and Yang energy if we look at Eastern Taoist traditions. An idea from that tradition is that the Masculine energy is the initiating energy, the more active energy and that the Feminine energy, as defined by this tradition, is more passive. Still, those types of views can reinforce the patriarchal view of what is Masculine and Feminine.

There is also a whole other way of looking at the term Feminine, which I was introduced to when I began studying Indian tantric tradition (which is very different from Western tantra, by the way), and this is that which is considered to be Feminine with a capital F.

Me: Awesome. I thought we would be heading down this path. Do say a bit more about this capital-F Feminine?

Cathy: Well, it is a context of what is referred to as non-dual as opposed to dual. Dual is where you are looking at two aspects of energy which we have in the space-time matrix. For example: day and night, we have positive and negative poles, and the way we are wired in our brains has Masculine and Feminine, male and female.

Going back to this non-dual tradition I mentioned, non-dual means 'not two', so they say there is not two, there is 'the one', like one source where all things arise from. Then, there is 'the many' which relates to all the differing forms. So, it's like each person is a unique expression of the one. The one being expressed in many forms. In this non-dual model, a model of oneness, we have everything created from consciousness and energy. It *sounds* like two, but consciousness and energy are, in fact, one. For example, the oneness consciousness is neither male nor female, it is simply The One. But people the world over personify energy and cosmic phenomena so that people can relate to and understand them. In this tantric tradition, The One is the energy that moves everything into form, which is like birth and this equates to the birthing of the universe. This birthing energy, I mean, of course, it has to be female. It is women who give birth on Earth, so the universal oneness energy which gives birth should be considered Feminine. In this sense, all energy and all power are Feminine. So, power is the Feminine.

Me: Makes sense.

Cathy: The Feminine is what gives birth to all life forms, and most indigenous traditions, pagan-type traditions, have always honoured the Feminine as clean and because of this, they honour the Earth. So, just by pure logical deduction, why would you not honour women? Why would you not put them on a pedestal as those that nurture life? Why would you not support that force?

The point of me talking about not just Feminine power or Masculine power as a two, but the Feminine as power is that it turns everything on its head for women. In patriarchal society, women are brought up witnessing power as *power over*, like force or domination, and power generally looks Masculine because in the past, most people in roles that wielded power were men. This is still the case today if we look at politics; yes, women are high-ranking politicians and heads of large organisations, but predominantly, it is male, or in the majority of cases, women have to present power in a masculine way in order to be able to compete and get ahead in careers.

The Feminine IS Power

Me: Whereas in this model you talk about, women and the Feminine are power. So, there is no competing with men required. Maybe women could stop competing with women as we are all the many expressions of this one force, the Feminine as power. I love this. It can help women get right with who we are: power. But not power over as an oppressive force; women are not going to go around trying to oppress men in the way that men have tried to oppress women because a power that does not need to compete would not have to do the oppression and control thing. I'd love to see a world where women are not destabilised by the curse of too much and not enough since they would know they *are* power!

You're right about leaders. Mostly we see males, and when we look at women leaders, certainly within politics, we see them unconsciously behaving in ways which are a kind of unbalanced masculine in nature, such as being forceful, single-minded, lacking compassion, inflexible and domineering (I am thinking of the previous UK Home Secretary. However, there is a chance though that she is not forced by the system into behaving abominably, but that she is simply evil), thanks to the male-favouring, male-dominated system they are operating inside.

It's no surprise that women can end up burned out and feeling really out of whack, bodily and emotionally, because the system such as it is – and let's call it that in big imposing capital letters, THE SYSTEM – is not one that is in any way nurturing or respectful to the Feminine as power.

Breaking Free on the Inside

Cathy: Yes. Patriarchy is an upside-down system. But if we just blame patriarchy, how do we turn it around? How can we heal from it? Take Joseph Campbell's model, the Hero's Journey, as an example of the human spiritual journey. In the Hero's Journey model, there are two stages; one is called The Meeting with The Goddess, the other is called The Woman as Temptress. We need to meet these aspects of the human psyche, our inner mapping, because there are plenty of people who do not view themselves as living under patriarchy in terms of their inner psychological make-up. They have broken free from it on the inside, to live with it in the outside world. We can take this Hero as not necessarily a male but as an analogy for the ego, and it is the sort of breakdown of the ego caused by the Feminine as the transformational force. It is the spiritualising force that transforms patriarchy into that paradigm where you have a framework of Oneness. You need something which can transform the shadow aspects of the Masculine (e.g., domination, violence, control and repression) and shadow Feminine (e.g., self-victimisation, helplessness, nagging, passive aggression, mistrust, trying to behave palatably to show you are not too much, or prove you are good enough) into their divine aspects and the Feminine is that force.

Me: Wow. This sounds like a way to healing through playing a game on patriarchy, like you said; breaking free from it on the inside to live with it on the outside. Oppression on the outside exists for sure in the world, and we can be activists against it through protest should we choose to, while on the inside, we can detangle from the patriarchy-inflicted wounds. We can rise up against the outer trappings of patriarchy, but we must turn our attention to healing our emotional landscapes from patriarchy too.

Coming Back to Earth

Cathy: One other way for women to heal is to put our attention on how we ground ourselves. All of this fear of being too much and not enough is connected with what some Eastern tantra calls the Earth Element Obstruction. People have a fear of being uprooted. What do we do in reaction to this? We find things to grasp onto for stability.

This grasping is shown in human behaviour as we try to accumulate more stuff, which we believe will stabilise ourselves, more money, more property, acquire more land and countries in an effort to show that the person is superior and not inferior. We live in a world where the Earth Element Obstruction is part of the fabric of life. We are not grounded.

Me: So women are trying to succeed in a world where the fabric of the system has evolved to make us feel ungrounded because, supposedly, the way to be sturdy is to prove you are enough and prove you have enough, vicious circle.

Cathy: To heal this seesaw between too much and not enough, we need to look at how we support, care for and ground ourselves without acting out the behaviours of the Earth Obstruction. I also think of a story from a Tantra tradition. Once upon a time, as all great stories begin, there was a great Goddess and a great demon. The great demon was very busy on Earth with his ideas of grandeur and power, busy conquering territories for himself. It got to a point where all of his armies had conquered all the territory and there was only one thing left that was not under his possession or control. That was the great Goddess. He had a plan. He decided to send her a marriage proposal, and this would mean that with marriage, the great Goddess would be under his control. Surprisingly, the great Goddess did not just tell him where to go. She said yes, I will marry you, but on one condition. You must defeat me in battle like you defeated everybody else. The Goddess turns herself into Kali, who is absolutely huge with a dangling tongue, and skulls around her neck and is ready for bloodthirsty battle. Kali defeats the armies and the great demon over nine days. On the eighth day, she has battled all the armies and the only two generals left are the main generals named Chanda and Munda, which loosely translated means too much and not enough. On the ninth day, she defeats the great demon himself. The moral of this story? There is no power greater than the Feminine.

Me: There is no greater power than the Feminine. Amen to that, I say! It's the Feminine also represented in a yoga text called the Devi Mahatmya when Goddess Yoganidra is called on by Brahma to wake Lord Vishnu so he can fight the two demons who are called too much and not enough. She needed to bring Vishnu back from sleep, restored, so he could fight.

Cathy: Yes, these stories are years old, but, I mean, what's changed?

Me: Hmmm, yes, it seems like old mythologies are being enacted. It's that human narrative of power gained purely for the sake of power.

How Do We Heal?

Me: The huge question in capital letters now is: HOW DO WE HEAL? How can women heal from the suffering of living under patriarchy if patriarchy is going to stick around for a while?

Cathy: When I work with clients, I walk them through the experience and understanding that a prevailing sense of awareness is within them. Against the prevailing state of pure awareness, we can dissolve wounded patterns back into wisdom.

Me: The power comes from the wound. Yes. I am seeing cross-over with the practice of Yoga Nidrā once again, because the state of yoganidrā is one where layers of personality, conditioning and beliefs can be dissolved or transformed. We can glimpse this state of pure awareness when we drop into the resting space of yoganidrā. Consciousness stays awake and there may be an experience or a tiny glimmer of being part of everything all at the same time, being non-dual.

Bring Up Your Wounds

Cathy: Transforming or healing can happen in pure awareness because the mind is less crowded. I want my clients to resolve the wounds which may have held them back from expressing aspects of themselves that want to be expressed. Working with women, it is really important to have this understanding of Feminine as power so we can start to unlock the wounding that is held by women, such as the fear of being seen.

Well, that was some real talk. Thank you, Cathy! We do need to bring our wounding into our awareness so that we may explore our true power, especially if we can source support from Wise Women like Cathy, who may hold space for us during the process. I know these explorations can be messy, but that is allowed. Plus, what else could we expect than mess after thousands of years being conditioned to forget our power?

She is Always There

There is power for us to turn to amongst the mess. The Feminine as power shows herself with so many faces. These faces are The One expressed as The Many, just as Cathy explained within the non-dual perception of life. The faces are the many faces of the Goddess. No matter where you are in the world, She is there. She warms our hearts with Her compassionate face as the Goddess Quan Yin from the Buddhist tradition. She rocks us with Her bone-jangling, wrathful, loving fury on the face of Hindu Goddess Kali-Ma. She asserts her freedom from the holds of patriarchy within Goddess Lilith. She engulfs us in romantic beauty as Greek Goddess Aphrodite. She catalyses our relationship with our wounds and shadow in the Sumerian tale of Goddesses Inanna and Ereskigal. She stands for the changes we cycle through as women, shown by the face of African Goddess Oya. She can be found on the sound of the forest wind as Roman Earth Goddess Diana. She keeps the comforting home fires burning in Her incarnation of Anglo-Saxon Goddess Frige. She is the originating divine spark within Sophia, the wisdom Goddess. Within the all-powerful archetypes of the Goddess, we also find the varied expressions of the power of womanhood. In case we hadn't already cottoned on to the fact that women are so powerful *because* of our many faces, this huge global pantheon of Goddess lore is yet another reminder that women are formed around the ever-changing anchor of our cycles along with our expansive potential for expressing power.

When we tell ourselves the story that we are not enough, we are limited by patriarchy's power play; we are stuck in the victimhood that patriarchy set up for us so long ago. We can instead choose what we say about ourselves, and this weakens the curse of too much and not enough. With practice, we can observe when we are mean and victimising toward ourselves. This observation is a key to freedom. We can turn toward kinder thoughts. When we are kinder to ourselves, resentful energy is released, making us feel lighter, more available and present for what we want to get up to in our lives.

The world is in a fucking state. Have you noticed? The ever-unfolding litany of corruption, lies, fascism, power grabs, elitist wealth transfers, medical restrictions that compromise rather than promote our health. My gut, no scratch that, my whole body tells me that we could do with calling on the Goddesses for comfort and power on the daily! She exists for us to call on when we most need Her to reignite or re-discover our inner power. The good news is that we don't have to reach too far or look away from ourselves to plug into the power of the Goddess to help the world to recover from its current state. Why? Well … let me remind you that you already have these many expressions of the Feminine as power, within the coding which makes you a woman. It was born into you through Sophia. Patriarchy has attempted to be the virus in our Feminine code long before our witches were burned. But unlucky for the patriarchal 'powers' that be, She was born into our blueprint aeons ago and She is not going anywhere. She knows that the exploits being played out on Earth are simply dramas which humanity must recognise, witness, untangle and rise up from.

She is expressed in the simplest ways. She is alive and well when we move our bodies purely for feeling good and for our healing, when we choose our most delicious foods, when we collaborate with like-hearted women, when we say *fuck no* because we really do mean no, when we allow ourselves to receive pleasure in any of its forms, when we honour the Earth, when we take time to honour our cycles, when value kindness instead of intellect, when we advocate for ourselves, when we adorn our bodies for joy not validation, when we scream into the night, when we give our kids a break, when we take to the streets, when we protect ourselves and our families from harm, when we fully recognise and respond to our needs, when we choose rest over busyness as usual, when we say *not in my name,*

when we no longer pour from an empty cup,

when we receive the wealth that we deserve,

when we remember we have nothing to prove.

In all these enoughness-empowered ways, we are alive as the Goddess because power is you and you are power. Not separated from power, at one with your own. We hold the power of ancient temple priestesses from many thousands of moons ago who sat sovereign in their enoughness. We hold the fragments of forgotten power in our blood, breath, and bellies. It is our soul-work to remember because when the women recover, the world will recover from patriarchy's power-hungry, paranoid fever dream.

Rising

What small (or larger) actions would you like to take that embody the Feminine as power? Consider the ways you move your body, how you carry yourself, the colours you enjoy wearing, how you adorn your body and environment, the rules you might dissent from, how you interact with people and yourself, the projects and communities you wish to create or maintain as areas where you might embody the Feminine as power.

Reflect on the creation stories you were told. How do these reflect the Feminine and Masculine?

Explore in writing or through artwork the difference between power and force.

Who or what have you given your power away to?

Where are the imbalances of power in your life? Consider familial relationships, work settings, intimacy, and in wider society.

Are there ways that you try to dominate people through force? What do you think might drive this need to be forceful?

Which of the Goddesses listed in this chapter do you resonate with? Do a deep dive to find out about this Goddess so you can honour her traits and energy in your life. If you do not resonate with any I listed, do an internet search for Goddesses from your culture or lineage. Check out the research of Megan Watterson or Uma Dinsmore Tuli as a starting point.

Create a sacred altar space in your home to honour the Feminine as power. Make it gorgeous and expressive. It can be as subtle or extravagant as you feel.

We need to call in the Feminine as power to awaken our enoughness so we can elicit change, because the people who run the world are at best, incompetent and at worst, psychotic. We might not know where to start, but we at least see the potential for rebirth from the destruction of antiquated hierarchical power.

She walked herself home.

Others followed.

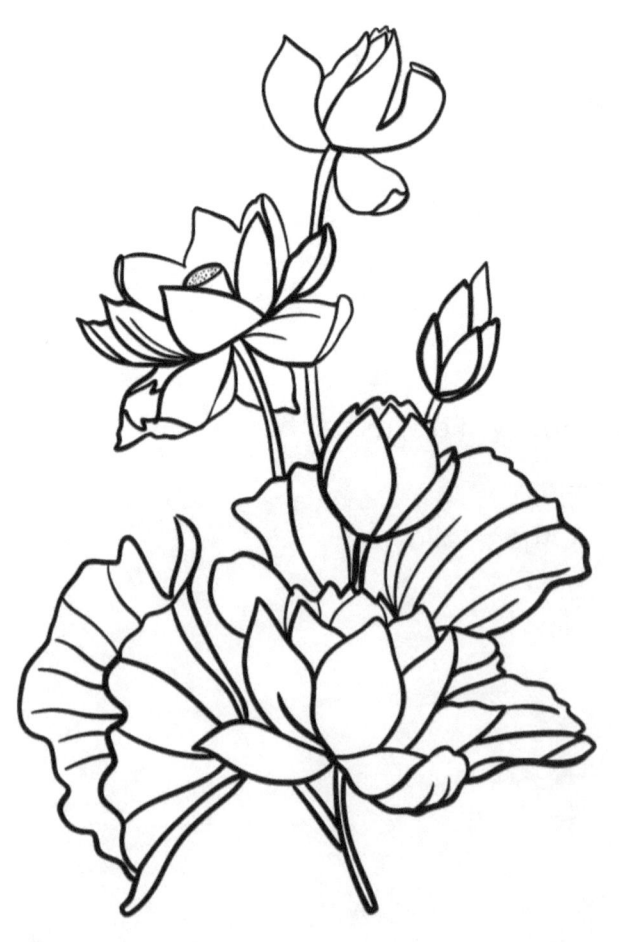

CHAPTER SEVENTEEN

Nothing To Prove

Rest

In this chapter's guided rest meditation, we are coming full circle, back to where we started, both closing and reigniting the circle.

Recover

Where do we go from here? The cycles continue.

When a woman reclaims the power of her enoughness, she awakens the recovery elixir for patriarchy's curse of too much and not enough.

Sounds good, so that should be it, right? Honestly, I thought I had those pearls of wisdom on lock. I had spent the majority of my life believing I was not enough, therefore, devoid of power. In the background of the moments when I did exercise courage, feeling the glimmer of power being restored, it was as if I would shut it off, thanks to the fear of being too much. If I started living as enough, would I be too much, too outspoken, too much of a boat rocker? I would feel the creeping pressure to get back in my invisible box, with invisible scold's bridal, with its own invisible shackles, locked shut until enoughness spoke to me once more.

Underworld

I wholeheartedly believed that telling myself I was enough would go some ways to healing the lifelong pain of not good enough. I think, on some level, telling myself the mantra *I am enough* did help me. I used to live like I was not enough, so it seemed to make sense to now make my life be about expressing my enoughness to show how far I had come. *I am enough* helped me day after day and will continue to do so. I wanted to prove I had made it back from my life as an addiction-prone, self-destructive younger me into a woman who was living as enough. I have indeed come a long way and made huge progress, but there was still a monkey on my back.

A few chapters ago I wrote that writing a book is a transformational process. This is because it is undeniably and inconveniently the case that the subject you choose to write about will come front and centre into your life like an attention-seeking Hollywood starlet desperate for the limelight. On the book journey, old wounds came up for more healing, wounds that I thought I had explored way back. Blind spots as dark as Inanna's underworld are revealed, hidden places made conscious in the light of new awareness. I thought it was only a coincidence that I had started having somatic experiencing therapy near the time I was literally shin-deep in notepapers, trying to organise my thoughts for this book. Of course, how could I write to women about recovering their enoughness without a deeper dive into my own metaphorical underworld?

Like I said, I thought I had it somewhat sorted; patriarchy's curse of too much and not enough could be dissolved when women reclaim their enoughness from the system which tries to oppress us. No matter how hard we try, patriarchy wants us screwed up, confused and powerless, chasing shadows to prove we are good enough for the world, for our relationships, our work, our children. Healing the collective wound of too much and not enough is the tipping point where we collectively catch our breath to regroup in empty space. A pause in the void. It is in the quiet of the void where wisdom arises.

I sat on my bed in a somatic therapy session. The collar of my t-shirt soaked in my tears while I was knocked sideways by the wisdom revealed from my own underworld. Being enough had become my compensation, the payment of the fictional debts I believed that I needed to pay for all the time I had spent fucking myself up. Being enough would settle a score with myself that I did not know I had been keeping, a grudge that I reminded myself of everyday. I had no idea that I was striving to prove my enoughness so I could escape entrenched shame for the mistakes I believed I had made: the eating disorder, the drugs, the men, the booze, the self-harm, the stress caused to my loved ones. If I could feel whole and live as enough while inspiring other women to find their version of enough, I would be able to pay off my karmic debt to the Universe. Pretty astounding for somebody who said that they don't believe in karma! My tears held the cleansing relief of self-compassion.

'All of this time, you have been trying to prove you have moved on and prove you are OK, because you thought you needed to make up for what you used to do to yourself. What if there is nothing to prove because you never did anything wrong? What if, given the circumstances, you were just doing the best you could?'

My therapist's words left me dumbfounded.

'If you could have done something else then you would have, but you were doing what you thought you needed to do to cope. You were only trying to survive.'

I sat in the void with my hot tears.

'There are no debts to pay.'

I had been trying to prove I was enough by being enough. It feels like some kind of Zen riddle. *Question: When is one who says they are enough, not believing they are enough? Answer: Anytime one is trying to prove they are enough.*

Doing our Bloody Best

So how do we reclaim the power of our enoughness in a world which devalues the Feminine as power? We could begin by entertaining the faintest possibility that all along we have been doing the best we could in the circumstances we have been in. You have been doing the best you can, and that, my friend, is enough. How does it feel?

You have nothing to prove, nothing to make up for. You deserve the peace that flows with the truth that you have been doing the best you could, and guess what, sometimes we get it wrong because we are human, not programmed machines. Doing our best isn't some shiny fantasy of tailored perfection. Our best might look like crying in a heap on the ground, downing sambuca shots to numb stuff out, or binging on biscuits, or starving yourself, or staying in bed for days, or quitting your job, or eating cereal for dinner, or not going to the gym, or saying *I'm not doing this anymore*. Sometimes the best we can do is to cope.

You are enough because you have been doing what you can. When we can do ourselves the huge service of getting off our own cases because we have been doing our best with what we have, the self-compassion of this realisation has the potential for an alchemical state change. We change from being in the state of proving and striving to the state of easeful receptivity, where we *feel* in our bones, blood, and bellies that we are enough. The feeling of enoughness stokes the fires for change. Our individual fires stem from the one Feminine power. And with this power, we can reimagine a new world, with new ways to live, if we can organise and take one right action after another.

She has never gone away. She values tiny steps as much as big leaps. She sees you, it does not matter if you cannot see her because power is in both the seen and the unseen. The benevolent Feminine Universal energy force which lives in you. She sees you are enough. You are She and She is you, always enough, just as you are.

Your debts are paid.

You have nothing to prove.

Rising

Reflect on what you have been trying to compensate for, or imaginary debts you believed you have had to pay. What have these debts felt like in your body?

Write them down, then burn them.

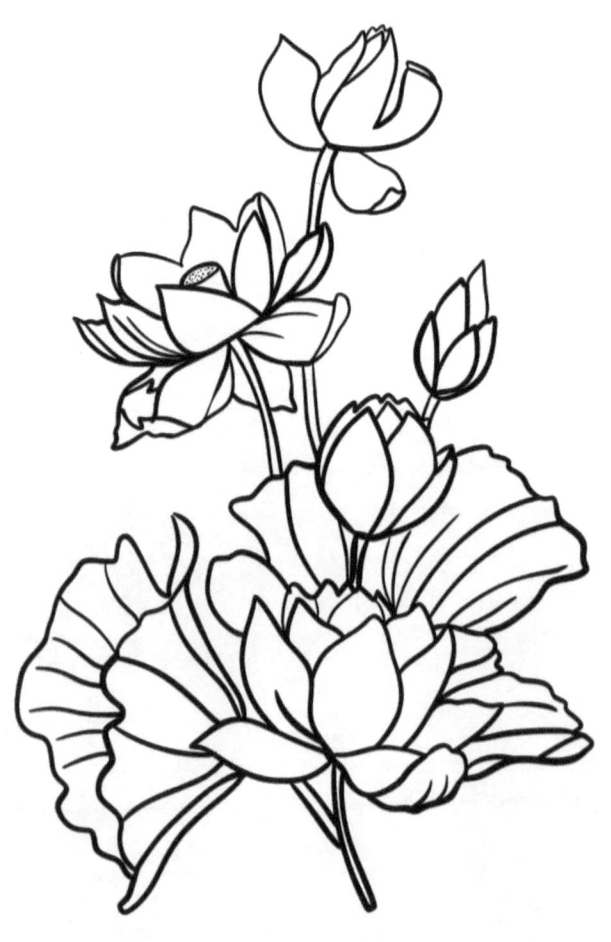

Parting Words: Living as Enough

I was worried that I did not have enough to write in this ending, where, for now at least, we part ways.

Uncovering and remembering our enoughness is an ongoing exploration. The most important thing we can do for ourselves is to step onto this path which will lead us home to our truth. What is the truth?

You are not too much.
Who you are is good enough.
You are enough.

Having spent some time practising Yoga Nidrā and rest during the journey of this book, I hope this has shown you a glimmer of the peace that is revealed when we dissolve and calm the mental patterns that are instilled by patriarchy's curse. Keep tuning into that quiet space because resting in the quiet will source your energy.

I'm also inviting you to join my You're Enough Yoga mailing list for vaguely regular reminders from me that you are enough, along with lovingly curated yoga wisdom. I'll look forward to sidling into your inbox!

Continue your path safe in the knowledge that you are damn fucking amazing, fully powerful and fully whole, and on the days when this feels like a lie, remember the biggest lies which have kept the Feminine suppressed for far too long.

It is a lie that you do not know power.

It is a lie that you are too much.

It is a lie that you are not enough.

You know your truth. Breathe it, own it, fucking live it.

Thanks for coming on this ride with me. We're always enough.
Love,
Sarah x

> *Enough! is dedicated to both of my grandmothers, the two Gwens, who both passed away during the completion of this book.*

Nowhere to get to

No thing to compensate for

No thing to prove.

Her heart relaxed.

Recovery Resources

If you are in a crisis (immediate harm from others or immediate harm from suicide), call your country's emergency services.

- Suicide Prevention for USA: https://suicidepreventionlifeline.org/ Tel: 988

- The Samaritans for UK: https://www.samaritans.org/ Tel: 0330 094 5717

- If you live in London and have suicidal feelings: Maytree Recovery House https://www.maytree.org.uk/ Tel: UK 020 7263 7070

Recovery from Sexual Violence

- The Havens: https://www.thehavens.org.uk/ 0203 299 6900

- Rape Crisis UK:https://rapecrisis.org.uk/ 0208 500 2222

- Rape recovery in the USA: https://www.rainn.org/ Tel: USA 800 656 4673

- Recovery book *Shadow and Rose: a soulful guide for women recovery from rape and sexual violence* by Sarah Wheeler https://www.youreenoughyoga.com/new-book-shadow-rose

Recovery from Addiction

- List of 12 Step programs for USA, for example, Alcoholics Anonymous, Over Eaters Anonymous, Gamblers Anonymous, Sex Addicts Anonymous: https://sobernation.com/list-of-12-step-programs
- List of 12 Step programs for UK: https://www.help4addiction.co.uk/12-steps-rehab-program-uk/
- You can also consult your regular doctor for help with substance addictions.
- *In The Realm of Hungry Ghosts* by Dr Gabor Matē
- *Soul Recovery* by Esther Nicholson
- *Dopamine Nation* by Dr Anna Lembke

Recovery from Abuse

- https://www.refuge.org.uk/ Tel: 0808 2000 247
- https://www.womensaid.org.uk/the-survivors-handbook/surviving-after-abuse/
- Trauma recovery (PTSD & CPTSD) :
  http://www.pete-walker.com/
  https://www.emdria.org/about-emdr-therapy/
- For counselling and psychotherapy in UK:
  https://www.bacp.co.uk/
- For counselling and psychotherapy in USA:
  https://www.betterhelp.com/
- *When the Body Says No* by Dr Gabor Matē

- Dr Ramani Durvasula (recovery from narcissistic abuse): http://doctor-ramani.com/

Eating Disorders

- BEAT: https://www.beateatingdisorders.org.uk/

Cult Recovery/Fundamentalist Religion Recovery

- *Combatting Cult Mind Control* and *Releasing the Bonds* both by Steven Hassan
- www.igotout.com
- https://www.tothinkagain.co.uk/
- https://www.daretodoubt.org/
- List of cults at https://culteducation.com/

General Mental Health (information on diagnosis and support)

- Mind.co.uk
- https://medcircle.com/

Coaching, Witching and Wisdom

- Rachel Smithbone: www.rachelsmithbone.com
- Bold Soul Coaching with Thea Anderson www.theaanderson.com
- Tom Pardhy, Life Coach: www.tompardhy.co.uk

- Natalie Farrell, Light Translator: https://nataliefarrell.co/
- Carol Cavalcante: https://thesoftbreezespodcast.buzzsprout.com/
- Cathy Rowan: Wise Woman's Journey www.catherinerowan.com

Burn-Out, Fatigue, Chronic Illness, Chronic Fatigue Syndrome and Stress Recovery

- https://www.charlottewattshealth.com/about
- For Chronic Fatigue Syndrome: https://drmyhill.co.uk/
- My websites: www.youreenoughyoga.com & www.reikirenge.com
- *Medicine Woman* by Lucy H Pearce

Further Reading on Gnostic Mythology

- *The Gnostic Gospels* by Elaine Pagel
- *Sophia's Tale* by Dr Sarah Walton

Notes

1. BEGINNINGS

1. https://www.priorygroup.com/blog/why-are-stress-levels-among-women-50-higher-than-men

3. FOUNDING FATHERS – HOW DID WE GET HERE?

1. 'Scared to be a Woman', *IndoctriNation* podcast
2. Starck, A., Stern, G., *The Dark Goddess*, Crossing Press, 1993.
3. https://www.ancient.eu/Kabbalah/

4. REMEMBERING OUR WITCHES

1. 'Traumatic Narcissism in Politics', *IndoctriNation* podcast

5. ENOUGH ALREADY: OWNING THE ALCHEMICAL PROCESS OF RECOVERY

1. https://www.sokaglobal.org/resources/study-materials/buddhist-study/thewisdom-for-creating-happiness-and-peace/chapter-3-14.html
2. https://www.wired.co.uk/article/china-social-credit-system-explained

6. REST IS A PATHWAY BACK HOME

1. http://www.pete-walker.com/fAQsComplexPTSD.html#recovering
2. https://rapecrisis.org.uk/get-informed/about-sexual-violence/statistics-sexualviolence/

7. ALLOWING IMPERFECTION

1. https://www.nationalgeographic.co.uk/science-and-technology/2021/05/endlessscrolling-through-social-media-can-literally-make-you-sick

8. BUSY GIRLS AND GOOD GIRLS

1. https://lesliesguidinghistory.webs.com/guides.htm
2. https://www.theatlantic.com/national/archive/2013/01/christopher-hitchens-onthe-mildly-fascist-founder-of-the-boy-scouts/272683/

9. BODY

1. https://www.theguardian.com/society/2021/jun/13/why-are-women-moreprone-to-long-covid
2. https://www.thelancet.com/journals/laninf/article/PIIS1473-3099(20)30568-5/fulltext
3. https://worldcouncilforhealth.org/multimedia/general-assembly-59/
4. Gilan, A., Laster-Haim, S., Rottenstreich, A., Parat, S., Lessans, N., Saar, TD., Dior, *The Effect of Sars-Cov2-BNT162B2 Vaccine on the Symptoms of Women with Endometriosis.* USA: National Library of Medicine, 2022.

5. https://elemental.medium.com/the-bizarre-and-racist-history-of-the-bmi-7d8dc2aa33bb
6. https://www.amnesty.org.uk/press-releases/yemen-detained-actress-and-modelrisk-forced-virginity-test

10. BLOOD

1. Tadros, E., *Reconstructions of the Coptic Church*. Ontario: McMaster University, 2015.

13. ENOUGHNESS FOR SALE

1. https://www.amnesty.org/en/latest/campaigns/2016/06/drc-cobalt-childlabour/
2. https://www.theguardian.com/commentisfree/2020/dec/01/amazon-workersfighting-for-their-rights
3. https://goodonyou.eco/how-ethical-lululemon/
4. https://www.theguardian.com/global-development/2019/oct/14/workersmaking-lululemon-leggings-claim-they-are-beaten
5. https://www.ilo.org/global/topics/geip/WCMS_614394/lang--en/index.htm

14. IT IS NOT ALL IN YOUR HEAD

1. *Who are the victims of domestic abuse?* Safelives.org.uk, Marac National Dataset, Bristol, 2014.
2. https://www.psychologytoday.com/gb/blog/somatic-psychology/201004/theconnections-between-emotional-stress-trauma-and-physical-pain

15. CULT

1. Hassan, S, The BITE Model of Authoritarian Control™, *Combatting Cult Mind Control: The Guide to Protection, Rescue and Recovery from Destructive Cults.* Freedom of Mind Press, 2018.

16. POWER

1. https://www.theguardian.com/society/2021/aug/17/my-bosses-were-happy-todestroy-me-the-women-forced-out-of-work-by-menopause

About the Author

Sarah Wheeler is an advocate for women recovering from the wounds of Patriarchy. She is a Reiki Teacher, Yoga Teacher, Author and founder of You're Enough Yoga in Hove, East Sussex. She is in her greatest joy when empowering women to uncover the medicine of deep rest and embodied movement revealing the truth of being enough; just as we are.

            youreenoughyoga.com
          youreenoughyoga@gmail.com

www.ingramcontent.com/pod-product-compliance
Lightning Source LLC
Chambersburg PA
CBHW030253100526
44590CB00012B/390